ADHD

Advance praise for this book

'Dr Prosser's book is a timely contribution to the ongoing debate about ADHD. By fearlessly tackling some of the thorny sociopolitical questions, he addresses issues that have been given far too little attention. In addition, his critique of the way medication is sometimes administered in the absence of a multi-modal approach should challenge all of us who work in this field to re-evaluate what we do.'

Rev Dr Peter Powell, Pastoral Counselling Institute, Sydney
and co-author of *Raising Difficult Children*

'As an educator, I am excited by Brenton Prosser's message about the social impact of having ADHD. His consideration of this issue will inform and empower both parents and teachers of children with ADHD in a number of ways. Firstly, the information provided in this book will help pave the way for positive relationships between teachers, their students with ADHD, and the parents of these students. Secondly, the book provides an alternative view of ADHD that will empower us as teachers to take up the challenge of using our knowledge and skills to develop pedagogical and interpersonal approaches that will allow students with ADHD to succeed in school. Finally, the notion of multi-modal support for these students through a whole-of-community approach would build a sustainable system able to result in greater positive outcomes for students with ADHD.'

Dr Kathy Baker,
Lecturer, Central Queensland University
and author of *Reading Success: A reading intervention for students with ADHD*

'This book is a great resource for all parents, teachers and health professionals who are dealing with ADHD. It contains helpful ways of handling ADHD behaviour, the types of treatment needed, and ADHD teenagers relating their own stories. It also explains how society and politicians are failing our ADHD children.'

Roslyn Mitchell
Secretary, Hyperactivity Attention Deficit Association (NSW)

'I warmly welcome Brenton Prosser's approach to ADHD. His emphasis away from a purely drug-oriented approach to a more multi-modal outlook is refreshing. I am sure parents of children with ADHD will find it informative and useful.'

Dr Antony Underwood
Paediatrician

'This book is easy to read, containing clear and concise information about ADHD. It covers history, assessment, treatment and educational advice, and is one of the few books on ADHD that actually reports Australian statistics. The author strongly emphasises the need for "systems" to change to fit the needs of the ADHD-er rather than vice versa. The chapter summaries provide the reader with the key points covered, and the case studies are an excellent way for parents and teachers to gain insight into the way young people feel about their ADHD. Most importantly, the book identifies that ADHD is not simply a medical diagnosis, and stresses the urgent need to recognise and manage the social, communication and educational deficits that result from ADHD.'

Susan Johnston, ADDults with ADHD (NSW) Inc,
member of the Learning Difficulties Coalition

ADHD

Who's failing who?

Dr Brenton Prosser

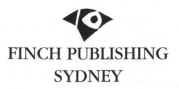

FINCH PUBLISHING
SYDNEY

To Cherie, Bob and Zac –
thank you for your patience, friendship and support

ADHD: Who's failing who?
This edition first published in 2006 in Australia and New Zealand by Finch Publishing Pty Limited,
PO Box 120, Lane Cove, NSW 1595, Australia. ABN 49 057 285 248

10 09 08 07 06   8 7 6 5 4 3 2 1

National Library of Australia Cataloguing-in-Publication entry

Prosser, Brenton James, 1970–
ADHD: who's failing who?

Bibliography.
Includes index.
ISBN 1 876451 71 8.

1. Attention-deficit hyperactivity disorder. 2.
Attention-deficit hyperactivity disorder - Diagnosis -
Australia. 3. Attention-deficit-disordered children -
Behavior modification - Australia. 4. Hyperactive children
- Education - Australia. I. Title. II. Title : Attention
deficit hyperactivity disorder.
618.928589

The author and the publishers wish to thank Paula Goodyear for her editorial input and creative
contributions to the manuscript during its formative stages.
Edited by Sean Doyle
Editorial assistance from Rosemary Peers
Text designed and typeset in ITC Garamond 10.5/14pt by J&M Typesetting
Cover design by Steve Miller – 154 Design
Cover photograph courtesy of alamy.com
Printed by Southwood Press

Notes The 'Author's notes' section at the back of this book contains useful additional information
and references to quoted material in the text. Each reference is linked to the text by its relevant
page number and an identifying line entry.

The names of all children, parents and schools mentioned in the book have been changed.

All Finch titles can be viewed at **www.finch.com.au**

Contents

Introduction

Joining a guided tour of the British Museum in London a few years ago, I skipped from one amazing ancient relic to the next, tracing the history of Western civilisation. Before long I found myself reflecting on Attention Deficit Hyperactivity Disorder (ADHD) and where it fits into human history. Walking over the polished floors, I wondered if having a biological propensity toward impulsiveness and overactivity would have been so bad if you were a Viking warrior, a late Renaissance explorer or a prolific painter. Then, peering into the staid glass cabinets and the ordered world of more recent centuries, I was also reminded that these behaviours would have been met with a stern rod in Victorian times.

It wasn't until several hours later, while sipping a dark English brew in a Paddington pub that it dawned on me how specific ADHD is to Australia, New Zealand and North America. Suddenly, the idea that each society and culture needs to find its own way of coping with ADHD made much more sense. In the United Kingdom that may mean more of a medical approach, to balance an overly sociological response to behaviours – but in Australia, New Zealand, Canada and the US it may mean the opposite.

It was from this realisation that this book grew. When I looked at ADHD from different angles, I found an environment where the competition for resources, arguments between professionals, political cost-cutting and media hype have all helped create a 'black and white' approach to ADHD. But this misses the point. The real battle isn't over the existence or non-existence of ADHD (where so many advocates expend so much energy) – it is over the deeper issue of who is responsible for planning a socially just response to the growing number of young people who do not fit society's expectations.

These are the young people who have difficult lives at school and for whom the very nature of ADHD limits what they can achieve. Through no fault of their own they struggle to meet the expectations of modern work and life, so their lives both at home and at school are increasingly troubled. Yet there persists a belief among many professionals, policymakers and popular opinion setters that somehow these children are the troublemakers.

❖

Do you ever feel like everyone is an expert on ADHD except you? Each day we read about ADHD in the papers, hear jokes on the radio, listen to popular songs about it or see children with ADHD on current affairs programs. Through these media we receive mixed messages. Should kids be on drugs? Do families get enough support? Is it just bad parenting? Why aren't teachers doing more? Have you heard about the latest cure for ADHD? Sometimes it seems the more you hear, the more confusing it gets.

This book is the product not only of my doctoral research project on ADHD but also of many years spent working as a youth worker, secondary teacher, political advisor, and now as a research fellow in education. Thanks to these experiences I have refined my thoughts about the many faces of ADHD. Hopefully, by sharing from these experiences in this book, I can help relieve some of the confusion.

If you want a quick fix for ADHD, then this is not the book for you. However, if you want to make informed decisions about how you can support your child/student with ADHD, then you will find a wealth of advice and ideas here. The book wades into the heated debate over the cause of ADHD and at the same time develops a compassionate, balanced and holistic approach to understanding the disorder. Along the way it includes discussions of ADHD definitions and diagnosis, drug use, adolescent accounts, the dangers of labelling, and the vital role of schooling and society. It also challenges some of the myths about ADHD. As such, it is the most comprehensive guide to ADHD written in Australia.

The main premise of the book is that if we ask only medical questions about ADHD, we will get only medical answers and more drug treatment. However, if we also ask educational, social and political questions, we will not only gain a better understanding of ADHD, but also possibly identify why drug use for the disorder has sky-rocketed in recent years.

Some people who are locked in the 'black or white' view of ADHD may feel threatened, and fear that I am trying to 'disprove' ADHD, but in fact in this book I am trying to do quite the opposite. By addressing some of the myths and misconceptions about ADHD, I want to encourage a broader view of ADHD that will be more useful in helping young people and their families. What I will offer parents and families, professionals and the public is a full and balanced view of a medical diagnosis that has become a well-known popular phenomenon. The core of my argument is that once we accept that some of our children are physically different in such a way that it causes them to fail at school and work (because of social preferences for certain behaviours), then we as a community need to decide how we will respond to that failure. I believe that leaving these challenges for doctors and drug prescribers to solve is effectively 'drugging and shrugging'; instead, we need to meet our collective responsibility to young people with ADHD and their families.

ADD or ADHD?

Before we go much further it is probably helpful to start by being clear about our terminology. This is one of the biggest sources of confusion about ADHD, and if you have heard about

ADD on the TV or the Net, you must be wondering, 'What's the difference?'. Put simply, ADD and ADHD are the two most recent versions of a medical label that's been evolving for over a century. The most common mistake people make is in thinking that ADD and ADHD are different disorders, with ADHD emphasising hyperactive behaviour. However, from a historical and medical point of view, these two labels refer to the same set of behaviours – it's just that one of them, ADHD, eventually replaced ADD as the latest medical theory. So the two labels can be used interchangeably.

This said, from a social perspective there are some advantages to thinking of them as separate labels. ADHD is a medical diagnostic category. It is the latest label for the latest medical theory. Yet ADHD has become much more than a medical theory in Australia. The growing public awareness of the disorder has made it part of popular culture – a well-known label for any bad behaviour in children. In this case it is often useful for clarity to refer to ADD as the public face of the disorder because it includes all the historical, media and social ideas or influences on young people and families – not just the medical 'ADHD'.

Where there *is* a difference between ADD and ADHD is in a lot of the hype coming from advocates, remedy sellers, drug companies, the mass media and the Internet. While ADHD is the official medical theory, ADD is more often the term used in the schoolyard or street to describe hyperactive behaviour. When people in the street use ADD they rarely make reference to the official diagnosis, but draw on popular culture instead. For this reason, I tend to use ADHD when discussing the medical theory of the disorder, but ADD when discussing its social and cultural implications. As for parents, teachers and professionals, it matters little which label we use so long as we remember that being labelled ADHD is more than a medical procedure – it is also a social process.

1

ADHD – myths and facts

'In his first year at school Ben learned nothing. He would get up from his desk while the teacher was talking, walk across the room and start colouring in on another child's work. Or halfway through a class he'd get up and wander into the playground to get a stick he'd been playing with and bring it back. He repeated Year 1 but he was still disruptive. Twice a week I was called into the principal's office. I was at my wits' end – I got to the stage where I was too embarrassed to walk into the school grounds. When he was seven, a teacher suggested I get him assessed by a paediatrician. The doctor thought he had ADHD and prescribed dexamphetamine. I was so stressed. I didn't want to put my child on speed.'

Mother of eight-year-old Ben

'James was hyperactive from birth and hardly slept. In preschool he simply couldn't sit still and listen to a story – he would just run around the room. At school, he was uncontrollable. Other mothers wouldn't speak to me – he'd taken off one child's glasses and stomped on them. It wasn't premeditated, he just didn't think. At seven, he was diagnosed with ADHD and started taking medication. He went from barely understanding the alphabet to reading fluently in 18 months.'

Mother of James, now 18

'When he was assessed for ADHD at 19 he walked out of the doctor's office, triumphant. He said, "I've got it. I've got ADHD...". It was as if he'd won a prize because it explained everything – why people thought he was crazy, lazy or dumb and why he couldn't do what the rest of the world could.'

Mother of Callum, now 25

Living with ADHD

Ben, James and Callum are among an estimated 80,000 Australian children and young people (most of them boys) diagnosed with ADHD. It is now the most commonly diagnosed childhood disorder in the US, and one of the most commonly diagnosed disorders in children in Australia. Since 1984, the number of Australian children using medication for ADHD has climbed by at least 26 percent, raising questions about its causes, diagnosis and the use of drugs to treat it.

These children's behaviour can have a major impact on their lives – it's usually hard for them to concentrate and pay attention, hard to sit still and hard to control impulsive behaviour that gets them into trouble and offends other people. When you're impulsive, words are out of your mouth before you've had a chance to think about their consequences; and you act before you think. Impulsivity can make a smart child look silly.

Problems like these reach into many different areas of these children's lives, making it hard to learn, to make friends and to be accepted, often bruising their self-esteem in the process. Children with ADHD are often sad – they don't set out to cause trouble and when they do, they feel sorry. And, unlike many other childhood disorders, ADHD doesn't attract much public sympathy.

Although one single term – ADHD – is used to describe the problem, it's actually a collection of three sub-types. There's the *hyperactive/impulsive* sub-type (meaning they're fidgety, excessively talkative, always on the go); the *inattentive* sub-type (meaning they're easily distracted, dreamy, forgetful, have difficulty following instructions and concentrating); and then there's the *combined* sub-type (a mixture of behaviours from the first two categories). As well as this, around 50 percent of children diagnosed with ADHD also have another disorder. The disorders that sometimes accompany ADHD ('co-morbid disorders' is their medical term) can include dyslexia, speech problems, specific learning difficulties, Oppositional Defiant Disorder (referring to children who are excessively aggressive, violent and confrontational) and conduct disorder (i.e. children who have trouble matching their abilities to the environmental demands placed on them). Some people would also add autism and Asperger's syndrome to this list, but this is still controversial.

Yet the fallout from ADHD goes much further than the effects on the children themselves. If you live with a child with ADHD or know someone who does, you'll know how much stress it can put on families; and if you're a teacher, you'll understand the daily juggling act of maintaining discipline and trying to meet the learning needs of all the other students in the class. Also, with increasing pressure on schools to provide more support for children with the disorder, and its over-representation in the health, welfare and criminal justice systems (it has been estimated that up to 25 percent of males in prison have ADHD), the disorder is becoming a broader social problem. ADHD has the potential to affect not just individual families but the community as a whole.

So how did we get to this point where thousands of Australian children need medication to manage their behaviour? At a time when our children should be in great shape, thanks to better health care and standards of living, why are so many of them affected by psychosocial problems like depression, anxiety, ADHD and other behavioural disorders?

Until now, our understanding of ADHD has come mostly from medical research, and this has contributed to the growth of prescription drugs as a first (rather than a last) resort for treating children with the disorder. After spending ten years researching ADHD and teaching children who live with it, I believe there's an urgent need to stop seeing ADHD as a **Why has ADHD emerged** purely medical problem with a medical **as a problem just in the** solution and start asking what other **last 20 years?** factors could be contributing to the situation. We need answers to questions that medicine doesn't have, like why is ADHD more common in North America and Australasia than anywhere else? More intriguing still, why is it that some Australian States have significantly higher proportions of children with ADHD than others? Why does ADHD affect boys more than it does girls – and why has ADHD emerged as a problem just in the last 20 years?

If we ask only medical questions about ADHD, we'll get only medical answers. That's why this book tries to understand ADHD by asking different questions – like what impact could our culture, our government policies or our social attitudes have on this disorder? While drug treatment can be important for treating children with the disorder, if we leave the problem of ADHD solely up to doctors and pharmaceutical companies, we are shirking our responsibility to nurture future generations of healthy Australians.

ADHD and me

I first came across ADHD in the early Nineties in South Australia when I worked as a coordinator for a respite camp for children with behavioural problems, like David.

Ten-year-old David turned up there one dark winter's evening – a small figure in oversized jeans and jacket who, according to the social worker, was suicidal, uncontrollable and likely to be the most difficult boy we'd encountered at the camp. He was also diagnosed with ADHD. David and I seemed to get on quite well, and in the quiet before the rest of the boys arrived at camp, I had time to show him around and help him settle in. So far so good – I was feeling relieved at such a good start. An hour or so later, things began to change. David became aggressive and violent, and demanded to be taken home. He missed his mum and didn't want to be around all these 'ADD kids'. As he began his 100-kilometre trek home from our rural retreat, we supervised him from a distance to see how far he'd go. He soon returned and, still angry, sat in the paddock until he cooled off.

The next morning was bright and sunny, and David appeared for breakfast, sleepy but cooperative. He seemed to enjoy the activities later in the day, but would approach a leader now and again and stress that he wouldn't be coming to the next camp because he didn't belong in a place with 'ADD kids'. He was, he insisted, 'normal'. 'Hypo camp' – his name for it – was no place for him.

David never did return to camp, and stories like his raised big questions for me, such as: how important are labels to children? Do we too often assume that kids just accept the labels we give them? How might they try to resist or redefine the labels that adults give them?

As it happened, I worked in these camps at an interesting point in the history of ADHD – by 1995, the number of new ADHD diagnoses in South Australia was on the up, and I noticed a dramatic change in the profile of the children sent to our respite program. While the camp had mainly helped families of underprivileged children in the past, social workers were referring increasing numbers of children with behavioural problems – in particular ADHD. As a teacher, I felt a mounting concern as I heard the horror stories these children told about school – so when it came to choosing a research project for my PhD, I jumped at the chance to study the impact of ADHD on adolescents in high schools.

It didn't take me long to find three trends with ADHD:

1. Research into the disorder focused on diagnosis and medical treatment, with little or no consideration of how labelling a child with ADHD might affect how they see themselves.
2. Treatment usually concentrated on the young person with the disorder, without checking for other factors in their environment that might be causing problems (e.g. post-traumatic stress, depression, family problems and even diet).
3. There was a keen media interest in ADHD but it rarely tackled the issue in any depth.

After my research, including many interviews with children with the disorder and their families, it became clear that there was a need for more social answers to persistent questions about ADHD – questions like, what is ADHD? What factors in a child's environment might contribute to the disorder or make it worse? How does ADHD affect the way children see themselves and the way others see them? What does ADHD tell us about us, the society that sticks on the label?

What is ADHD?

It's around 3 p.m. on Friday afternoon in a below-street-level Parliament House office in Adelaide, where I'm working as a consultant on ADHD to the South Australian Democrats political party. I'm gazing upwards through the window, watching the feet of people walking past on King William Street – and putting off the moment when I have to deal with my list of 'ADHD phone calls'. Eventually, I decide I can't postpone it any longer and dial the first number.

'Mrs Smith? Hi, my name is Brenton Prosser, I'm returning your call.'

'Dr Prosser ... thanks for calling back. I heard you interviewed on the radio yesterday and wanted to tell you about some recent research that proves the existence of ADD.'

'Which research is that?'

'Well, I'm not sure. I just saw it on a video last week, showing how the ADD brain is different, and I was concerned that you'd said on the radio that ADD didn't exist ...'

'That wasn't exactly what I was saying; I think what I actually said was that we don't have a test yet to prove who has ADHD ...'

'Well that's why I am calling – you should have a look at this video because it shows scientific proof that ADD exists. My two sons have ADD and I think my husband does too, but he won't go to a doctor to be checked. I just get really upset when people get on the radio saying ADD is not real and blaming parents. It is real, and I have to live with it every day.'

'I never said it was because of poor parenting, I just said that we need to be clear about what we know about ADHD and what we don't know.'

'Well maybe not, but comments like that don't help. My kids' teachers don't believe in ADD and they treat me like I'm a troublemaker because I go in to defend my kids. My kids are the ones that get picked on by others, especially the eldest. All kids get up to stuff, but it's always my kids that get blamed and have to go to the principal and then I have to go and sort it out ... people getting on the radio and saying that ADD doesn't exist don't know what it's like ...'

I left calls like this until last thing on Friday because they were usually so demanding. Unlike the mother in the conversation above, many people who called knew little about ADHD. Some would blame it on television, while others would say ADHD occurred because children were deprived of attention. More often than not, the calls came from parents (and sometimes teachers) desperate to help a child. I found this most difficult, especially when they pleaded with me to provide a quick solution – but there is no quick fix.

ADHD's many contributing factors

From these conversations with parents and teachers, I began to realise how many differing opinions there were about ADHD. As far as medicine is concerned, most researchers now agree that the symptoms of ADHD (i.e. persistent hyperactivity, impulsivity and difficulty concentrating) are caused by a subtle difference in the parts of the brain that manage behaviour, concentration and self-control, while some believe it is a neurological disease (though the evidence for this is still inconclusive). Yet there's more to ADHD than just what is going on in kids' bodies. Let's go one step further and look at the social factors that influence ADHD.

Even with a difference in the brain that causes certain behaviours, it's also true that how acceptable – or unacceptable – certain behaviours are depends a lot on the attitudes of those around. For instance, being hyperactive or impulsive wouldn't necessarily have been an disadvantage for a gladiator, an explorer or a pioneer – but it can be a real problem in a twenty-first century classroom, not to mention in a Western way of life that's more and more about sitting down rather than moving around. Just think for a minute how much of our lives now involve inactivity: we sit down in cars to travel short distances that past generations would have walked, cycled or ridden on horseback. Many of us sit down to work, and in our free time we sit to watch television and DVDs or use the computer. When we shop, unless we do it – seated – via the Internet, we drive to the mall, where escalators take us up and down, saving us the trouble of being active.

Instead of just asking how children with ADHD are failing in our society, we should also be asking what it is about our society that's failing them

When we remember that many health problems are a combination of genetics and environment, this inactive lifestyle has important consequences. For instance, you may inherit a tendency to put on weight – but if you're working eight hours a day in the fields in rural India, living on rice and lentils, you're unlikely to develop a weight problem. On the other hand, if you work in a call centre and eat fast food, you could easily become obese. It may be that in some children ADHD develops in a similar way – that is, it happens when normal inherited human qualities like the tendency to be overactive collide with a way of life that's becoming increasingly inactive.

Some parents have difficulty accepting that there may be factors other than just physical problems underpinning ADHD. This is because there's a common assumption that if your body causes a problem it's somehow more 'real' than a problem caused by social or environmental factors. Yet to better understand ADHD, we need to ask questions about both its social and its biological aspects. We need to ask ourselves if the problems it causes are only problems because of the values that exist now, in the early twenty-first century. At different times and in different places through human history, the behaviour we now call ADHD would not have presented the problems it does today. In an era when work meant burning up physical energy on a farm or in a workshop rather than sitting at a workstation using your head, I wonder if hyperactivity would have made any headlines at all.

'Hyperactive' heroes

Journalist Jonathan King (from the *Sydney Morning Herald*) tells the story of when Australia's longest-surviving World War One veteran Peter Casserly (who died in 2005) was at school in the early 1900s. Casserly loathed 'book learning' so much that at 13 he defiantly buried his schoolbooks in a park opposite the headmaster's office. He then left to become a blacksmith's apprentice. After joining up at 19, Casserly went on to survive the Western Front and was later awarded a medal for bravery for rescuing a swimmer who'd got into difficulties.

Another 13-year-old who ran away from school, Frank Hurley, became one of Australia's greatest photographers. He accompanied Douglas Mawson on a pioneering trip to the Antarctic in 1911 and later documented the horrors of the Western Front in World War One.

These men are not rare examples. Most of us have in our family histories a story of a relative who just did not fit into school but made their way in the old days with energy, creativity and hard work. One can only ponder that if Casserly and Hurley were 13-year-olds in a twenty-first century school today, would we have them assessed for inattention, oppositional behaviour and over-activity? Or, as American ADHD expert Dr Lawrence Diller reflects: 'I worry about an America where there's no place for an unmedicated Pippi Longstocking or Tom Sawyer.'

It seems to me that what we now call a disorder could be blamed at least partly on a mismatch between the natural diversity of human behaviours and a world that has changed so much in the last 30 years that these behaviours no longer fit. This isn't to dismiss the difficulties families face, but to point out that as a community we all need to take some responsibility for the growing ADHD crisis. Instead of just asking how children with ADHD are failing in our society, we should also be asking what it is about our society that's failing them.

But this is not to say that *all* influences from the environment or society are behind ADHD. Let's have a look at the main myths and misconceptions surrounding ADHD and replace them with facts.

Myth: ADHD is caused by too much television and poor nutrition

Fact: This is definitely not the case, despite what you see on television. While recent UK research, for instance, has found that children who eat fresh, unprocessed food and have access to water have better concentration and are calmer and more alert in class, that's not the same as having ADHD. While it's also true that some children are sensitive to some substances in food (including some additives in processed food as well as chemicals in natural foods), this doesn't mean they have ADHD. If you're worried about a child's behaviour, and these factors might be the problem, it would make sense to check their diet or have them assessed for any food intolerances by a hospital allergy unit before getting them checked for ADHD.

Myth: ADHD is caused by poor parenting

Fact: This is a gross overstatement and an over-simplification. Although poor parenting can make it harder for children with ADHD to develop the social skills they need for school and adult life, poor parenting – like diet – is an influence, not a cause. And while poor parenting may cause ADHD-like behaviours in some children, these can be improved by teaching parents better parenting skills. But when a child has ADHD, the problem will continue with even the best of parents.

Yet the myth of the bad parent is very persistent and can make life for families of children with ADHD harder still. Parents of ADHD kids often describe how they feel judged by other parents and hurt by these claims. The ordeal of dealing with an unruly child in public day after day is bad enough without the condemnation of other people. Current affairs programs that present sensational stories of out-of-control children and powerless parents don't help either. What doesn't make such dramatic viewing – and therefore gets less airtime – are the lives of deeply committed parents with great parenting skills struggling to do their best. And the sad irony is that the conscientious parents are the ones who come under fire for trying to get the best for their child at school: many are labelled 'complaining parents', reinforcing the notion that a 'problem child' is a reflection of a 'problem parent'.

The stress that ADHD can cause for families can't be emphasised enough. Poor parenting may not cause ADHD, but it can make good parents look like bad parents. Even perfect parents (if they exist) would struggle with the demands of ADHD. Instead of being used as a stick for beating parents, ADHD should justify more compassion and support because the challenges are so much greater.

Myth: Parents can just drug their kids

Fact: Medicating your child is a major decision for any parent, and I've never met one who took it lightly. Psychostimulant drugs for ADHD don't cure the problem but they can improve the symptoms. Many parents, like those of Ben and James at the beginning of this chapter, eventually try drugs out of desperation, and the dramatic change in their child soon convinces them. Others ask if it's possible to treat their child without drugs.

Those who decide against drug use argue that a child can have the symptoms of ADHD but be treated successfully with non-medical approaches that teach skills to improve memory and concen tration. Meanwhile, those who opt for drug use often say their child's behaviour problems are so severe that only medication can help him or her cope. Both views are legitimate, depending on the child, but in practice, it's rare for children diagnosed with ADHD not to be on medication. The reason behind this is simple. ADHD is a medical diagnosis, and with it comes access to prescription medication that is not otherwise legally available. So, if you don't want your child to use drugs, having him or her assessed for ADHD isn't all that helpful – it's more useful to work on strategies to improve problem behaviours rather than getting a diagnosis that provides you with a treatment you don't want.

The decision to consult a doctor and possibly have your child take medication for ADHD is daunting. On one side is the fear that your child is falling so far behind at school that it may affect his or her future, and the hope that medication can help your child be 'normal' and learn important social and academic skills. On the other is the controversy over medication prescribed for ADHD. With illicit drug use now a major problem among young people, some parents worry that if their children use prescribed amphetamines it may increase the risk of addiction to illicit drugs further down the track.

What benefits do drugs offer for ADHD?

Psychostimulants, the drugs that treat ADHD, are drugs that stimulate the brain. The two main psychostimulants used to treat ADHD are the amphetamine dextroamphetamine (or dexamphetamine) and a similar drug called methylphenidate (or Ritalin).

Dextroamphetamine and methylphenidate work by stimulating those parts of the brain that help control hyperactivity and impulsivity. Since the chemical make-up of these two drugs is different, one may suit one child better than it may suit another.

It's important to realise that the prescription dose of amphetamines in prescribed medication is much smaller than anything sold on the street. The best comparison I have heard is that if ADHD medication were cannabis, you would need to smoke something the size of a street-light pole to get a proper hit. When a character in the TV series 'Desperate Housewives' says she takes her son's ADHD medication to keep her 'zippy', it's at best a placebo and strictly entertainment.

For children and young people with ADHD, these drugs have several benefits. Not only do they improve concentration and self-control in most children, but by making it easier for them to concentrate they provide an opportunity for them to learn important academic, social and organisational skills. This can do a lot to boost their self-esteem, which in turn can help them do better at home and school.

The side effects of medication

The main side effects of the medication are a tendency to cause insomnia and suppress appetite; it can also cause stomach pains and nausea. While insomnia is more of a short-term problem, the effect of low appetite over a number of years can affect a child's growth. Other risks tend to be social – like the possibility that children come to believe that a drug is responsible for their behaviour, rather than their own decisions. However, teachers and families who are aware of this can work to minimise this risk. Some children – though not all – also feel there's a social stigma that comes with taking an otherwise illicit drug for medical reasons.

Some parents worry that drug use will increase the chance of their child becoming addicted to drugs, but there's no evidence that ADHD medication leads to greater drug use in either adolescents or adults. If anything, my research suggests that the experience of taking drugs legally for ADHD takes away the thrill of illicit drugs, makes young people better educated about their risks, and therefore more determined to avoid amphetamines as adults. In the minds of young people with ADHD, amphetamines are more commonly associated with failure and difficulty than with having fun. If young people with ADHD go on to use illicit drugs, it's more likely to be because their behaviour has made them feel alienated, rather than any addiction to their medication. My research found little evidence of drug dependence – instead, most children want to try life without medication in their teens. Most young people were more interested in fitting in and making friends than in taking amphetamines.

If you're considering medication for a child with ADHD, perhaps the most useful question for parents should be, is medication your first or last resort? Few parents in my research knew there were any treatments available other than medication. This is a real concern given that medication isn't meant to be the frontline approach for ADHD, but just one part of a broader 'multi-modal' approach tailored to the needs of the child. This approach includes not just medical support, but also psychological, educational, social skill and family support.

Medication doesn't fix the problem, it only provides an opportunity to intervene

If you've tried a range of strategies and therapies with little success, then the benefits of medication use may outweigh its disadvantages. So if medication is currently your first or only line of treatment, then it may be wise to do more homework – consult an educational psychologist and a dietician, for instance, to rule out any other issues that might be a cause of problem behaviours or be making them worse. Medication, remember, doesn't fix the problem; it only provides an opportunity to intervene. To paraphrase a colleague of mine, Professor Robert Reid

– a specialist in ADHD from the University of Nebraska – 'pills don't make skills'.

Myth: 'It's not me, it's my ADHD'

Fact: While working at the respite camp, I noticed that when boys were told off for some reason, they often came back with, 'It's not my fault, I have ADHD'. What this showed me was that children with this disorder are like any other child – they test the limits and make excuses. The difference, of course, is that children with ADHD have the added complexity of a label associated with challenging behaviour. In some ways, it's good to see young people not passively accepting a label and using it to suit their own needs. It can lead to things like asking for more time to finish an assignment or better advocating for their needs.

Yet they also need to learn the difference between appropriate negotiation and avoiding responsibility. A recurring comment from young people in my research was that medication did not make them behave properly – it just made it easier to choose how to behave. No child wants to be labelled 'deviant' or 'disabled', but when they're faced with one failure after another it's understandable that some children try to salvage some dignity by blaming the less stigmatised term 'disorder'.

Parents, teachers and others involved with children with ADHD can help with this by not raising the bar for success too high. In other words, they need to create situations where the distance between a child's ability to behave and what is permitted is not so great that he or she constantly fails and needs to use the label as an excuse.

Myth: 'We all have ADHD'

Fact: Another common perception of ADHD is that it's just an extreme version of normal behaviour and that we all have the potential for 'ADHD moments'. Every child goes through stages of hyperactivity, impulsiveness and inattention – it is part of normal development. You only need to look at a toddler at the 'terrible two' stage or at a class of 13-year-olds on a Friday afternoon to wonder what normal behaviour is. The process of growing up – which includes learning how to behave appropriately – is different for every child. What separates ADHD behaviour from what we all experience at different times is that:

- it causes a child to fall behind the 'normal' rate of development; and
- it causes significant problems for them socially, including at school or work.

The faster pace of our lives can push us all towards impatient, hyperactive, impulsive and inattentive behaviours. The pressure to perform and compete keeps increasing, working hours are longer, and information technology – once predicted to bring more leisure – means we're expected to produce results faster. Television and computers have also changed the way we think, encouraging shorter concentration spans and activities that tend to shut off the outside world and the kind of human interaction that helps us learn about appropriate behaviour and develop life skills.

We bring our children into, and expect them to cope with, this world – a world where the workloads of both adults and school students are increasing to meet the expectations of success in Western societies, and where the amount of free time spent outside school and work to let off steam and be creative is shrinking. We're all under pressure from twenty-first century living, and many of us have worked out our own ways to control hyperactive, impulsive and inattentive behaviour, or at least to find a good outlet. However, children with ADHD are unlikely to be able to do this without considerable support. The extreme nature of their behaviour pushes the boundaries of what's acceptable in modern society. When someone confronts the parent of an ADHD child and says that 'we're all capable of having ADHD sometimes', they should remember that not all of us face life with these behaviours *all the time* – and that's the difference.

Myth: An ADHD child is a problem child

Fact: Many people, including some teachers, claim the disorder is just another name for problem behaviour – the only difference with ADHD is that behaviour has been allowed to become more extreme. Some argue that this extremity is due to the inadequacies of parents and the difficulty of dealing with the behaviour in the modern classroom. In the past, 'problem' children were usually ignored or punished. Today, they're more likely to be under the care of the medical profession because of the current trend toward defining childhood problems as disorders to be treated by doctors or psychiatrists.

Meanwhile, some opponents of medical explanations for behavioural problems suggest that a medical diagnosis is just a ploy to get children to the front of the queue for resources and a 'cop-out' for parents. These people argue that we should treat disorders such as ADHD like any other behavioural problem.

Yet what's worrying about considering ADHD as just another name for 'problem kids' is the implication that somehow this makes it less of a problem. Does a problem only become real when it has a label like ADHD? Do we now have so many needs but so few resources that we have to distinguish between 'real' and 'fake' problems? Have we set the bar for empathy and support so high that having a problem is no longer enough to justify compassion and help? We should not be dismissing the needs of our troubled children, whether they have the ADHD label or not. We should be helping parents to help their kids with ADHD.

What should parents do to help a child with ADHD?

Parenting isn't easy at the best of times. Having a child with hyperactive and impulsive behaviour is harder still, so it's no surprise that parents want practical help for their child as quickly as possible. In this chapter, I have tried to explore some of the questions that initially face parents considering ADHD. In the next few pages, I want to take this one step further by providing ten practical tips to help you as a parent make sound decisions both during diagnosis and while trying to negotiate support from your child's school.

10 tips for parents on diagnosis and school support

1 Try not to have your child diagnosed and treated with drugs before the age of seven. While some doctors argue for early treatment to minimise problems, this has led to children as young as 18 months being prescribed drugs for ADHD. Remember that development varies greatly between children in their early years. If you're concerned about your child's behaviour, use the time before seven to try non-drug approaches that might help. This could include using rewards to teach organisation and concentration skills, or asking the teacher to seat the child in a place where there are fewer distractions. Involving your child in more tactile learning approaches and giving them the opportunity for creative and energetic outlets will help. You may also wish to consult some non-medical professionals such as nutritionists, school psychologists, counsellors and tutors who can help with diet, communication skills, anger management, organisational skills and alternative ways of learning. Remember, drug treatment should be the last resort, not the first.

2   Just because a child improves with drug treatment doesn't prove he or she has ADHD. All children respond to amphetamines in the same way – it's just that the impact is more noticeable in children with hyperactive behaviour. If you think your child has ADHD, make sure the diagnosis is thorough and that the doctor consults not just you, but also teachers and others who care for your child. Beware of doctors who either make a diagnosis or change levels of drug use over the phone without assessing your child in person.

3   Ask your doctor about multi-modal treatment – that is, the use of other non-drug strategies to improve your child's behaviour and skills. It is recommended internationally as the best treatment for ADHD. Using drugs alone is a bit like treating high cholesterol levels only with medication, instead of with better diet and more exercise. Multi-modal treatment can include a range of therapies and approaches such as behaviour management, remedial tutoring and teaching social skills to help the child relate better to others (see Chapter 2 for more about this). Ask the doctor how he or she plans to help you develop a multi-modal strategy. Your child needs this approach to help prepare for the increased social and academic demands of secondary school. If your doctor doesn't know about multi-modal treatment or argues that drugs are enough, find another doctor.

4   Don't confuse your child with his or her behaviour – just because a child behaves badly doesn't mean he or she is 'bad'. Healthy self-esteem is vital for the development of all children, and those with ADHD may end up hating themselves because they find it hard to behave themselves even when they want to. Try to reassure your child that they are loved for who they are, not what they do. This helps build the child's self-esteem and improves the chances of success.

5   Encourage your child to think of taking ADHD medication as a way to help them make the right choice. Help them to realise that they are still the ones making the choices; the drugs just make it a little easier. Don't let them blame everything on ADHD – instead, remind them that even children on medication can choose to misbehave.

6   Most young people should not take medication for more than three years – by that time they should be making good progress with their multi-modal treatment. Think of this period of drug treatment as a time to help your child develop the skills needed to succeed at school and later at work. As your child matures, it will be their ability to use the skills that they learnt during their drug treatment that will determine whether ADHD troubles them as an adult.

7   Have regular breaks from drug treatment – one weekend a month or even once a week if you have good support. Try not to be scared of these times; try to use them as an opportunity for your child to demonstrate his or her newfound skills. Plan these breaks for times when there are few distractions and little family stress – and don't expect too much too soon.

8   Build strong relationships with your child's teachers. This is often difficult because the priorities of parents of children with ADHD and teachers can be at cross-purposes. Teachers are often in the unenviable situation where they have to choose between meeting the great need of the few or the general need of the many. If you can support your child's teacher (rather than attacking them for not doing enough) there's a better chance of your child getting the help they need in the classroom.

9 If things don't work out at school, keep a paper trail of notes from meetings and phone calls, making sure you record the time, place and the names of all the people involved. Too often, parents have legitimate concerns about school responses or feel that their child is being singled out but have only their memory to support their claims. It then becomes the school's word against the parent's – often resulting in a long stalemate. This can make things worse for your child because schools sometimes label the parent as a problem and, instead of seeing your child's needs as legitimate, blame the 'problem parent'.

10 Remember that the ADHD experience will give you and your child a good understanding of the disorder – don't underestimate your own expertise.

These are just a few basic tips for parents who are thinking about their child and life with an ADHD diagnosis. In the following chapters there will be more advice, strategies and insights into ADHD that will help you make informed decisions with your child for the future.

Key points

- ADHD is among the most commonly diagnosed childhood disorders in Australia.
- It is not caused by poor parenting but it can make the best parent look poor.
- If the problem is sugar or TV, then it's not ADHD.
- Changes in Western society in recent years have made life harder for active and impulsive people with short attention spans.
- There is much more to ADHD than just drug treatment.

2

An epidemic of ADHD or over-prescription?

'We make no claim to knowing all the answers to the
problems of ADHD. We do, however, claim to be able to
distinguish between what we know, what we think we
know, and what we do not know. And many assumptions
pertaining to ADHD fall into the second and third
categories.'

Professor Robert Reid, US ADHD expert

Over the last decade, most ADHD treatment in Australia has
been by the medical profession – and during this time the
use of drugs for ADHD has grown dramatically. Yet while medical
research tries to improve diagnosis and drug treatment, there's a
lot about ADHD that it can't explain. For instance:

- Medical research knows that children with ADHD are children who have significant problems at home, school and work, but doesn't have a scientifically proven test to show who has ADHD and who hasn't.
- Medical research knows that all children respond to psycho-stimulants with increased attention, but doesn't know why or how.
- Medical research suspects ADHD is genetic, but can't explain how much of the problem is due to nurture, not nature.
- Medical research suspects that there are problems with mis-diagnosis, but doesn't know how widespread this is.
- Finally, medical research knows that drug use for ADHD has sky-rocketed in the US and Australia over the last 15 years, but cannot fully explain why it's happened in these particular countries.

This last point raises a few questions. Is the high level of drug use in Australia and the US due to softer standards for diagnosis? Does the recent rapid increase in diagnosis mean more children have the disorder or is it that there's less support available to help them cope? Why are so many parents accepting the use of psychostimulant drugs to treat their children?

US research found that parents have their children tested for ADHD only after becoming frustrated with the lack of support in schools. If this is true, it puts medical specialists in a very difficult situation. Telling desperate and distressed parents that 'there is little they can do' goes against why most people choose to become doctors. US ADHD specialist Dr Lawrence Diller, author of *Running on Ritalin*, remembers this exchange with a worried mother.

'Doctor, do you test for ADD?'
My first conversation with Sheila Gordon, the mother of six-year-old Steven, began with this question. It is a question I first heard only a few years ago, but today hardly a day goes by without a concerned parent raising it. Her voice uneven with

distress, Sheila went on to tell me that Steven, her only child, was struggling in the first grade and that the teacher advised having him tested for ADD.

Confronted with a familiar dilemma, I shifted uneasily in my chair. How could I tell Sheila over the telephone that, to my knowledge, there was no real test for ADD? Perhaps she would think that I wasn't well informed about the condition – after all, the teacher told her to get Steven tested. I wanted to tell her that an ADD diagnosis is complicated, and that the condition now described as ADD can have many causes and symptoms.

I understood Sheila's anxiety about her son. I had heard the same note of distress over the phone from many parents, and I've seen the pain and havoc that a seriously unhappy, acting-out child can cause in families. Medication might be part of the eventual treatment, I said – but I would never recommend it as an option before seeing the child.

The causes and consequences of ADHD

The strongest belief among medical researchers is that ADHD is caused by a neurological problem that triggers hyperactive, impulsive and inattentive behaviours. What this means is that a part of the brain is not working properly, so that a person is on the go, acts without thinking and is distracted to the point of causing problems at home, work and school. It's also thought that genetics may play a part in especially difficult cases, but so far no-one has found a gene or DNA link for the disorder.

ADHD also affects children's ability to develop the social skills that help them make friends and keep them

As if disrupting home life and making it difficult to learn aren't bad enough, ADHD also affects children's ability to develop the social skills that help them make friends and keep them.

A classic example of this problem is in the story of John, a gangly 14-year-old who agreed to take part in my research. He'd been diagnosed with ADHD two years earlier and his parents had tried a year without medication before trying Ritalin. They'd seen some improvement in his behaviour but not in his ability to concentrate. His social and organisational skills weren't strong and his homework was chaotic. Yet what troubled him most was his difficulty making friends.

'I don't really have any friends at school any more,' John told me in one interview.

'Why do you think that is?'

John didn't look up from under his mop of sandy hair, but his response was quick and to the point. 'Because I can't really trust anybody – because there are some people who say they'll be your friend but what that really means is that they'll be your friend when there's nobody else around.'

'But you've had friends before?'

'I had other people as friends, but 'cos I like joking around I started to annoy them even though I didn't mean to.'

I waited, hoping that silence would tease out more information.

'Like with one friend, I kept going on about some computer game being better, you know something like that, and I was starting to get on his nerves. And, yeah, he got a little mad but I'd keep talking and talking ... and most of the time I just wouldn't notice he was getting mad. Recently I've been noticing it more, the signs of somebody who is getting angry. It's hard to keep friends.'

John's story highlights one of the main concerns that children with ADHD talk about: the difficulty of making friends and the fear of being treated differently. But these aren't the only consequences for children with ADHD and their families. Others include not just difficult behaviours, but also criticism from other parents and the ever-present concern that the child will fail at school and be unable to get a job.

Another example is the story of 13-year-old Michael, told by his mother, Sarah.

'Michael's adopted. I don't know if he told you that … and we found out all his family history. He has two cousins who have ADD. His mother has ADD and his birth sister who lives with another family has ADD.'

Sarah paused. Realising she was nervous about being interviewed, I asked her how old Michael was when they adopted him.

'Michael was two days old,' she said. 'If he wasn't sleeping he was always on the go, and I thought it was normal because he was my first …'.

'… and you had nothing to compare it with', I said, trying to be supportive.

'Yes, well … when he started at school I realised something was wrong. Anyway, we got him tested and he did have ADHD.'

Knowing that many children with ADHD are diagnosed shortly after starting school, I probed a little further about the move from home to school. 'So was it causing problems at home or were things fine at home and it was just the school that made you realise something was wrong?'

'It was school,' said Sarah. 'It was the pressure he was under at school and the pressure on me too. We got a phone call every single day when he was at school.'

Searching a little further, I asked:

'What sort of relationship did you find …?'

Sarah interrupted '… with teachers?'

'Yes, with teachers first and then with the other parents,' I said.

'Other parents were real hard because it was Michael who'd

run like crazy in other people's houses and they'd go, "Why can't you control your child, why don't you smack him?". But you can smack and smack and smack and it doesn't do any good. So it was hard for him to make friends when he was younger, and it was hard for us as a couple to make friends. People didn't understand … you know, they saw this normal child on the outside. If he'd been handicapped on the outside then it would have been different, but he's not, he's handicapped on the inside.'

Returning to the first part of the question, I asked: 'And teachers – how did they respond?'

'Up until he went to the new middle school, they didn't.'

With children spending about half their daylight hours at school, ADHD is a major part of many of today's classrooms. Doctors and other professionals work with children with ADHD for only a few hours each month, while teachers – like parents – are in the frontline, and their support is vital in helping students.

Yet teachers, often lacking the resources and training to help them cope with ADHD, are in a difficult situation. When confronted daily by struggling students and anxious parents, and especially if they have no school support, they might do what the teacher did in Lawrence Diller's story. This directs parents who are unable to afford other approaches to ADHD to rely on bulk-billing doctors and subsidised medication for help.

Methods of diagnosis

Currently there's no simple test to prove a child has ADHD – instead, doctors use a checklist of behaviours to diagnose the disorder. There are two versions of this checklist. The one used in Europe and the UK is from the World Health Organisation's (WHO's) *International Classification of Diseases (ICD-10)* (see Appendix A for more information about this); while the other – used in Australia, New Zealand and the US – is from the American

Psychiatric Association's *Diagnostic and Statistical Manual of Mental Disorders*, or *DSM-IV* (see box below).

The main difference between the two checklists is that under the WHO version, a child's behaviour needs to be more extreme to qualify for a diagnosis – this results in fewer children being diagnosed. The *DSM-IV* looks for six or more behaviours from the two lists below that have lasted for six or more months at an abnormal level. To qualify for a diagnosis of ADHD, some of these behaviours need to have appeared before the age of seven. They also must be causing problems in at least two different areas of his or her life (e.g. home and school). The two different lists help diagnose which of the three sub-types of ADHD the child has. As mentioned, these are:

1 inattentive sub-type (once known as Attention Deficit Disorder);
2 hyperactive/impulsive sub-type; and
3 combined sub-type (meaning the child has behaviours from both lists).

The *DSM-IV* checklist

Inattention
- often fails to give close attention to details or makes careless mistakes in schoolwork, at work or in other activities;
- often has difficulty sustaining attention in tasks or play activities;
- often does not seem to listen when spoken to directly;
- often does not follow through on instructions and fails to finish schoolwork, chores or duties in the workplace (not due to oppositional behaviour or failure to understand instructions);
- often has difficulty organising tasks and activities;
- often avoids, dislikes or is reluctant to engage in tasks that require sustained mental effort (such as schoolwork or homework);

- often loses things necessary for tasks or activities (e.g. toys, school assignments, pencils, books);
- is often easily distracted by extraneous stimuli; and
- is often forgetful in daily activities.

Hyperactivity/Impulsivity
- often fidgets with hands or feet, or squirms in seat;
- often leaves seat in classroom or in other situations in which remaining seated is expected;
- often runs about or climbs excessively in situations in which it is inappropriate;
- often has difficulty playing or engaging in leisure activities quietly;
- is often 'on the go' or often acts as if 'driven by a motor';
- often talks excessively;
- often blurts out answers before questions have been completed;
- often has difficulty awaiting turn; and
- often interrupts or intrudes on others (e.g. butts into conversations or games).

However, there are some questions as to how accurate this list is as a way of measuring ADHD. One concern is that the use of checklists is subjective, not objective. This means that too much is left up to the personal views of each doctor, which lacks the certainty of a blood test or an X-ray. There's also a growing concern that other causes of similar behaviour could be mistaken for ADHD. These similar causes include conduct disorders; anxiety; obsessive compulsive disorder; post-traumatic stress; learning disorders; substance abuse; and depression or other disorders.

To help Australian practitioners use these checklists more effectively, the National Health and Medical Research Council recommends they ask for educational assessments and look at other factors that could shed light on problem behaviour. These factors include the child's:

- medical and psychological history, as well as the family's;
- physical and neurological health;
- developmental stage;
- behaviour in both home and school settings; and
- language development and academic performance.

These guidelines came about because of concerns about inappropriate diagnosis. Government departments and parliamentary inquiries into ADHD have raised similar questions – and with good reason.

One afternoon, I was talking to 12-year-old Billy, one of the younger students in my study. He wasn't being too cooperative – until I asked him about his doctor. Billy had been on medication for some time, but still clearly remembered being diagnosed. He had been seeing a Dr Wilson and, almost without thinking, Billy told me, 'He swears a lot.'

'Why is that, do you think?' I asked.

'He's trying to identify with me,' Billy replied candidly. 'He's the best doctor, I reckon.'

'Well what did he do ... how did he test for ADHD?'

Billy's response surprised me, but I've since come to be less surprised – I've heard so many stories like it. 'He gave me dexamphetamine and said "Take this". So I took it, and I could concentrate, and it was fine, so I thought it was a good idea.'

To clarify that Billy hadn't just forgotten, I asked: 'He didn't try other sorts of stuff?'

'No.' Billy responded with a tone that suggested it was an odd question to ask. 'So how did the medication help?'

This was a better line of questioning from Billy's perspective and he quickly explained the benefits of drug treatment. 'It's just hard to sit there and do your work ... it's weird. But when I have the tablets they make me work and do as much as I can. Like, I write and write and write and write ... but if I don't take them, I do four lines and then think, "What am I doing this for?". I suppose it doesn't really take the ADHD away, it just gives you the ability to choose to work.'

Drug treatment

Billy's description highlights why psychostimulant drugs are the best-known treatment for ADHD. They can have a dramatic and life-changing impact, an observation backed up by many teachers and parents, including Margaret, a high school teacher who told me how amphetamines had radically transformed one of her teenage students, Ben.

'I happened to go down to the library and there was Ben doing a project. He was so focused,' said Margaret. 'When I asked the librarians how long he'd been there, they said he'd been there for 40 minutes. I went over and said, "Ben, c'mon, is this some joke?" "No", he said, but when I asked him how he was feeling, he replied, "Really strange."

'Once he began taking the medication, the first few weeks were amazing, and he still had better concentration even when he'd got used to the drug. But years of misbehaving had given him a "misbehaving habit" and it eventually started kicking in – I think he just missed his old behaviour patterns. So I put him on a subject lesson check and by then he had the Behaviour Management Support Unit in. He seems to have levelled out now, and there are whole lessons now where I forget Ben is there – I can get on with dealing with other students. He's even up to date with his work.'

While methylphenidate (Ritalin) is used more in the US, dexamphetamine has been used more in Australia – probably because it has been the psychostimulant available at a subsidised cost through the Australian Pharmaceutical Benefits Scheme (PBS). This is a point reinforced by New Zealand having a significantly higher use of methylphenidate when both drugs are subsidised. In New Zealand, both methylphenidate and dexamphetamine have been eligible for government subsidy – although the laws changed in 2002, due to high levels of methylphenidate use and concerns about illicit use. Now a special authority is required from the Ministry of Health for this subsidy.

However, the situation changed in Australia in August 2005 when it was announced that methylphenidate would be included in the PBS. Previously, the Australian Federal Government had considered including Ritalin in the PBS, but negotiations with its manufacturer over price had not been successful. It will be a matter of great interest to ADHD advocates and researchers to see if the New Zealand experience is matched in Australia and there is a growth in methylphenidate use, especially among low-income families now that the drug is subsidised.

Although medical research has shown that these drugs can result in improved concentration and reduced activity without major long- or short-term side effects, it can't explain why stimulant medication helps slow children down. A common theory is that ADHD happens because the parts of the brain that manage behaviour, concentration and self-control are underdeveloped and don't work efficiently. Using drugs to stimulate these parts of the brain to work effectively helps the child to concentrate and behave better. This is often called the 'paradox effect', because while you'd expect stimulants to speed children up, in fact they slow them down.

The scientific study that's often used to support the theory of the 'ADHD Brain' was by researcher Alan Zametkin and colleagues at the National Institute for Mental Health in the US. His 1989 preliminary study found that glucose – the brain's major fuel – was used differently in the brains of *parents* of a hyperactive child. However, not only were the study's methods criticised, it was only a preliminary study and hasn't been duplicated since – in other words, it hasn't met the criteria of good scientific research. What's more, Zametkin never claimed that the results proved that there was a different type of brain with ADHD, nor that there was a genetic link with ADHD. This hasn't stopped a wide range of advocates and authors saying that Zametkin's study is proof that the brains of kids (and not their parents!) with ADHD work differently.

It is precisely because there is no ADHD brain to cure that most authorities agree that drugs should be one of a range of interventions

Another myth about ADHD is that if drugs can help children with ADHD, it must follow that ADHD medication can be used for diagnosis. In other words, if the child behaves better on medication, doesn't it mean there is something there that is different? If only it were that simple – but a crucial study by Judith Rappaport in the late 1970s gave psychostimulants to hyperactive boys as well as to boys with no behavioural problems. The study found that psychostimulants had the same effect on both groups. While this didn't disprove the possibility that drugs can stimulate an underdeveloped brain, it did disprove that the brains of children with ADHD work differently. In short, if a child responds to drugs, it doesn't prove they have ADHD – only that they are a child.

One of the challenges with both the Zametkin and the Rappaport study is that their findings are now more than 20 years old. Quite rightly, people may ask why science hasn't provided more recent information on the relationship between psychostimulants and hyperactivity? Well, the simple answer is that it has tried, but it faces some restrictions. Firstly, the principles of ethics that guide research have improved significantly, and increasingly restrict tests with unknown consequences for human participants. Secondly, there are problems getting a control group together to compare the impact of drugs. Or, to put it simply, if you were a parent of a child without hyperactivity, would you volunteer your child to try psychostimulants for the sake of science?

The current consensus among evidence-based scientific researchers is that all children respond to stimulant medication with better concentration and less activity, but young people with ADHD respond more dramatically because their difficulty is greater. As children mature and their bodies change, these areas of underdevelopment 'catch up', and the impact of medication changes, becoming more like that of adults. It is precisely because there is no ADHD brain to cure – and drugs only provide a 'window of opportunity' – that most authorities agree that drugs should be one of a range of interventions for ADHD.

This view, however, is not without its critics, as was demonstrated in recent research from the National Institute of Mental Health in the US. This suggested that medication was more effective for ADHD than behaviour modification or community support, and that the combination of treatments didn't make much difference. There has been a lot of criticism about how this study was done and, again, the findings haven't been duplicated since. Still, this does nothing to stop the belief that drug treatment alone is enough to treat ADHD.

> As Billy explained: 'I kept going to Dr Wilson to get my medication, and I was also going to Dr Jones – he's a child psychologist – but I think Mum stopped sending me to Dr Jones because she didn't think I was telling him anything ... I mean, he was just asking questions and I was answering the best I could, but I don't know if they were the answers he was looking for.'

Growing drug use

It's hard to know just how widespread ADHD really is. While figures show a dramatic growth in drug use for ADHD in Australia, they only tell us how many drugs are prescribed – and not how many people use them. Nor do we know the exact extent of ADHD elsewhere, because different countries vary in the way they diagnose ADHD and measure drug use.

Internationally, drug use across ten Western countries grew on average by 12 percent between 1994 and 2000. The US and Canada used the most, with Australia and New Zealand in equal third place. Australia and New Zealand used significantly more drugs per head than the UK, Sweden, Spain, the Netherlands, France or Denmark. With the exception of South Africa, there is little drug treatment of ADHD in Africa and Asia. Before 1998, however, there was little drug use anywhere except Australasia and North America. In 1999 Australia and the US were the only two countries to be warned by the United Nations about their excessive use of psychostimulants to treat behaviour disorders.

The period of most dramatic growth in Australia and the US was the early 1990s. Between 1990 and 1995, drug use for ADHD in the US more than doubled to include around 2 million children, while drug prescription rose by 480 percent. During the same period, drug use in Australia grew by around 500 percent with the amount of drugs prescribed growing just over 700 percent. If one considers only dexamphetamine, the number of prescriptions grew 2400 percent between 1991 and 1998, while Ritalin prescriptions grew by 620 percent. Much of Australia's growth in this period was a case of 'catching up' with American trends that had started in the mid-1980s.

The growth in Ritalin use in New Zealand started a few years later, but between 1992 and 2003 prescriptions rose from just under 3000 to almost 70,000, while dexamphetamine prescriptions grew from less than 1000 to around 5000 in the same period. Notably, these figures would suggest a link between government subsidy and levels of use, as dexamphetamine is subsidised and used more in Australia, while in New Zealand both drugs are subsidised and the use of Ritalin is much more prevalent.

Another factor in Australia and the US is that drug use for ADHD isn't spread evenly across the country. Drug use varies hugely from one State to another. Prescriptions in Victoria increased 20-fold between 1988 and 1994, with a seven-fold growth between 1992 and 1995. Growth in NSW was slightly slower over the same period. Between 1991 and 1997 there was an estimated 50-fold increase in psychostimulant prescriptions in South Australia for children with ADHD, but it's Western Australia where drug use grew most rapidly:

Growth in PBS prescriptions dispensed for dexamphetamine sulfate, 1993–2003

	NSW	Vic	Qld	WA	SA	Tas	ACT	NT	Australia
1993	9 127	2 475	3 659	5 623	3 128	257	302	107	24 678
1994	17 312	5 045	6 083	11 338	5 264	813	689	238	46 782
1995	29,276	9 844	9 885	18 466	7 828	1 853	1 267	625	79 044
1996	39 800	15 001	14 988	29 009	12 397	2 760	1 688	677	116 320
1997	46 708	19 525	20 099	39 036	15 832	4 252	1 838	671	147 961
1998	52 905	25 305	23 296	49 880	18 157	5,314	2 038	663	177 558
1999	58 863	30 401	27 074	60 437	19 539	6,878	2 363	858	206 413
2000	62 788	33 207	31 298	68 869	18 236	8 303	2 886	762	226 349
2001	61 433	33 572	34 102	75 185	19 089	9 075	2 967	785	236 208
2002	62 743	32 950	35 927	81 892	19 130	9 271	3 143	735	245 791
2003	61 390	32 422	36 362	86 980	19 585	8 790	3 188	708	249 425
Total	502 345	239 747	242 773	526 715	158 185	57 566	22 369	6 829	1 756 529

So one thing we do know is that drug treatment for ADHD leapt significantly in Australia in the 1990s. When looking at this and the following table, it is important to note that these figures only cover the growth in dexamphetamine (which was PBS-listed) and not methylphenidate (Ritalin), which is also used for ADHD.

Number of PBS prescriptions dispensed for dexamphetamine sulfate, 2003

State/Territory	Number of prescriptions	Population	Number of prescriptions per 1000 population
New South Wales	61 390	6 716 277	9.1
Victoria	32 422	4 947 985	6.6
Queensland	36 362	3 840 111	9.5
Western Australia	86 980	1 969 046	44.2
South Australia	19 585	1 531 375	12.8
Tasmania	8 790	479 958	18.3
Northern Territory	708	198 700	3.6
ACT	3 188	322 579	9.9
Australia	249 425	20 008 677	12.5

While trends in most States seem to have flattened out since the turn of the century, these recently released figures still show relatively higher levels for some States, which continue to raise eyebrows. For instance, the number of prescriptions in Western Australia remains around four times higher than the rest of Australia and is more than ten times higher than the lowest number, in the Northern Territory.

Multi-modal (i.e. non-drug) treatments

In theory, all children with ADHD should have what's called multi-modal treatment – a 'treat the whole child' approach. Depending on the child, this could involve:

- *Psychological approaches* which can help children improve problem-solving skills and self-control; anger management training, behavioural training and group therapies.
- *Educational approaches* which can include new learning strategies, improving writing skills, consistent behaviour-management strategies, remedial tutoring, self-esteem activities and individual education plans.
- *Other therapies* which can include speech therapy, family therapy or social skills training, and teaching the child how to interact with others in a more appropriate way.

Although these therapies are available, they're not always afford-able or accessible – because they can involve so many different health professionals, they can be very expensive. So, although the multi-modal approach is recognised as the best – it is recom-mended by the National Health and Medical Research Council, Australia's peak health advisory body – in reality there's more emphasis on medical care, because drugs are relatively less expensive than other treatments. Also, in Australia poorer fami-lies can access subsidised medication, and visits to doctors can be subsidised by Medicare. For this reason, most families have their children assessed for ADHD because diagnosis is the only way to get affordable treatment – even though this may not be the best or most desired treatment.

Dubious alternatives

Surprisingly, most families in my study were not aware of non-drug treatments. However, just like medical therapy, there are question marks over some alternative therapies. While I was advising the South Australian Democrats party on ADHD, I often met 'solution sellers' lobbying politicians to endorse treatments. These included supplements like anti-oxidants and amino acids that claimed to reduce the need for ADHD medication. On one occasion, someone sought support for vegetable-based 'gummy bears' that he claimed cured ADHD because these children were not getting enough vegetables. On another, I met a representa-tive from a company selling another non-drug therapy for ADHD; she wanted details of families I'd interviewed in my research so she could contact them in a direct marketing campaign. When I explained that I was bound by a code of ethics to keep that information confidential, she urged me to think about how much commission I'd get from each sale if I'd just cooperate!

Parents need to be careful with alternative approaches because not only are there some questionable practices, there is also some questionable research. Many presume an understanding of ADHD that we don't have. For a group to claim that a lack of nutrients or insufficient oxidation of the blood at birth are to blame, it needs the support of solid research which – as yet – doesn't exist. My experience of alternative treatments is that instead of having good scientific research to support them, there's usually a collection of Internet sites endorsing their claims, some testimonials from families whose lives have been transformed by the treatment, and a small body of research, usually by the 'expert' selling this particular therapy. I am yet to find an advocate of an alternative treatment who can explain how their therapy works and support it with good research.

Having said that, some alternative treatments may help some children with hyperactive, impulsive and inattentive behaviours – but I must stress that this doesn't mean they cure ADHD. Having these treatments help is totally different to suggesting a new cause of ADHD that these alternative treatments can fix. If alternative treatments do remove the symptoms, then ADHD may not have been the best explanation in the first place. It is always best to consult your doctor about any treatments that your child may be using.

The other concern I have with some alternative treatments is that they often echo the 'pills not skills' approach of drug treatments. Simply to swap a non-drug intervention for a drug intervention still misses the important psychological, environmental and educational treatments of the multi-modal approach. As my work with teenagers revealed again and again, when only drug treatments are used in the primary school years, the risk of significant problems increases with the greater social and academic demands of secondary school. While drugs (or non-drugs) may help break the behaviour cycle, they're no substitute for social and educational interventions. And if this principle is true for drugs, why should it be any different for alternative medicines?

Misdiagnosis and overdiagnosis

Many people ask if the recent rapid growth in drug use to treat ADHD means the disorder is being overdiagnosed. In other words, they are asking if children with milder forms of ADHD (who could probably cope with psychosocial and educational support alone) are being labelled ADHD and given medication needlessly.

What makes answering this question difficult is that, due to diagnostic shortcomings, we have no way of telling how many children have ADHD, so how can we tell if there are too many? What we do know is that there are very few young people legally allowed access to these drugs without an ADHD diagnosis. So it's fair to assume that most of the rapid growth in drug treatment is a reflection of more children being diagnosed with ADHD. On the other hand, because we only have diagnostic checklists (rather than an objective test for ADHD), this leaves open the potential for well meaning doctors to diagnose according to their beliefs about ADHD or their desire to help struggling families. In short, we don't know how many of those diagnosed have ADHD.

We don't know how many of those diagnosed have ADHD

Even the experts disagree on how many kids have ADHD. In the UK, levels have been estimated as low as one percent, while estimates in the US have been as high as 23 percent. Usually, estimates in Western countries fall in the range of three to five percent. This is true of Australia and New Zealand, where the commonly accepted figure is three to five percent of school-aged children.

If we accept the most used figure of around five percent, it seems unlikely that overdiagnosis of ADHD is occurring. Drug use for ADHD stands at less than three percent of children in the United States, and between one and two percent in most Australian States (with WA over four percent). If ADHD were overdiagnosed, you'd expect rates consistently above five percent. While prescription rates might be high in some parts of Australia, there's no evidence that this is nationwide. In all probability, then, diagnosis and drug use in Australia is not the crisis it is sometimes made out to be.

Yet, while overdiagnosis is unlikely, there's little doubt that misdiagnosis happens here, in New Zealand and in the US. By misdiagnosis I mean young people being labelled and given drugs for ADHD when this is not the most useful treatment. The reasons for misdiagnosis can include:

- when other causes of similar behaviour are confused with ADHD (these can include mild cases of autism, Asperger's syndrome, Tourette's syndrome, Language Learning Disorder and Oppositional Defiant Disorder);
- the limitations of diagnostic tools (when well-meaning errors are made because diagnosis is left up to the judgement of doctors rather than via an objective 'physical' test);
- sloppy diagnostic practices (on rare occasions some doctors do not follow the checklist, and diagnose over the phone or without properly checking a number of environments); and
- when overzealous medical practitioners are too eager to get a particular diagnosis (such practitioners explain their higher level of diagnosis by being 'ADHD experts' who are leading the field of medicine).

There is no real way of knowing how many young people are misdiagnosed and little evidence to support conspiracy theories against doctors. Yet, given the number of different ways a child can be eligible for ADHD under the *DSM-IV* checklist, misdiagnosis is a very likely possibility. When misdiagnosis occurs, it is bad news for those both with and without the condition. Drugs may help children who do not have ADHD with their behaviour in the short term, as they affect all children in a similar way.

What is worrying is if the true cause of their problems goes undiagnosed – then they're not getting the treatment they really need, which is likely to get better long-term results. As for those who really do have ADHD, misdiagnosis is no help to them either. Well-publicised examples of dubious diagnoses can imply that their problems aren't really caused by ADHD.

Misdiagnosis hides the real issue behind the growing number of young people diagnosed with ADHD, namely that there are many families in real need. The fact that so many families go looking for an ADHD diagnosis tells us that they've had no luck with education and other support networks. The situation suggests we need to find out more about how much support is being provided and if a lack of support for families is behind the growth in ADHD.

So is there currently an ADHD epidemic? The answer is probably not – but how can we be sure without more information and more accurate testing? There is still a lot less that we know about ADHD than what we don't know or only think we know.

Key points

- Asking medical questions about ADHD produces only medical answers – and more drug use.
- No-one knows what causes ADHD.
- There's no objective test to prove a child has ADHD – instead, doctors use a checklist of behaviours to diagnose the disorder.
- If a child responds to drugs it doesn't prove they have ADHD – it proves that they are a child.
- While every ADHD diagnosis is an individual one, the huge explosion of ADHD in the Nineties was more than the sum of its individual parts.
- Claims of an ADHD epidemic are overstated.

3

The evolution of ADHD

'The mainstream definitional platform now accepted by a majority of professionals, social institutions, parents and the public is fairly simplistic: ADHD is understood as a genetically inherited, biologically based mental disorder in which dysregulation of certain brain chemicals causes affected individuals to have problems with paying attention, controlling impulsivity and regulating motor activity.'

Dr Katherine Ideus, US ADHD researcher

How did medical science discover ADHD and – more fascinating still – how did something that was once an obscure medical diagnosis develop such a high public profile? Let's take a look at the social and historical background against which ADHD evolved, and at the controversy that's made it the hot topic it is today. The scientists may have set the ball rolling, but thanks to the combined influence of the media, the Internet and popular opinion, ADHD has developed an identity of its own that most scientists would scarcely recognise.

A history of the label

What we now call ADHD has worn a number of different labels over the last century, and behind each new label was a medical theory. The word 'theory' doesn't necessarily mean something isn't real – rather, it's saying that this is the best understanding we have at a particular time.

1900

ADHD's origins go back to the UK around the turn of the last century (though some people suggest that the idea of difficult behaviours being caused by a brain syndrome first emerged in 1854). The person most often linked with the birth of medical theories for hyperactive behaviours was a British paediatrician called, ironically, George Still, whose research linked brain injury to unruly behaviour. He argued that overactivity and the lack of self-control were moral faults caused by damage to the brain through poor nutrition, injury, disease, or inherited traits.

This theory wasn't subject to much public scrutiny at first – but even if it had been, few eyebrows would have been raised at the idea of linking poor morals with brain injury or underdevelopment. This is because Still's research coincided with a time when science and philosophy in England were heavily influenced by a movement called Social Darwinism.

Although not part of Darwin's theory of evolution, Social Darwinism applied the idea of survival of the fittest to the development of human societies. It argued that Europeans were socially more civilised and technologically more advanced because of their superior physical traits. In that period of history it wasn't uncommon to believe that the shape of your head could show if you were intelligent, that lumps in certain places on your skull determined your chances of being involved in crime, and that dark skin colour made you prone to immoral behaviour. One reason why these ideas gained so much acceptance was because they gave pseudo-scientific support for the push of European nations to colonise other countries. It was similar thinking that had earlier enabled English colonists to declare Australia *terra nullius,* and that was later adopted by the Nazi movement to justify their annexing of Europe. It's hard to overestimate the impact of Social Darwinism on the thinking of the time – it certainly influenced George Still but, more importantly, it meant that few questions were asked about how credible his medical theory was.

The 1920s

The next stage in the development of the ADHD theory came on the heels of the worldwide encephalitis epidemic in the early 1920s. This viral infection of the brain, caused by a new and persistent strain of influenza that first emerged in 1918 (which some contemporary commentators have likened to the recent outbreak of bird flu), left many children with behavioural and psychological problems that attracted medical research. The breakthrough came when two US researchers, Hohman and Ebaugh, noticed similarities in the over-activity of children who'd survived encephalitis and that of people who'd survived head injuries from World War One. Consequently, a new medical theory emerged – Organic Brain Damage.

The 1930s

A flurry of medical research into the brain, much of it aiming to find ways to relieve severe headaches, led – by accident – to one of the most important early developments in the treatment of Organic Brain Damage. Working in a US encephalitis clinic in 1937, Dr Charles Bradley experimented with an amphetamine substance to increase blood pressure and relieve headaches. To his surprise, he also noticed an improvement in the behaviour of the people he treated – and this is how drug treatment for hyperactive behaviours was born.

The 1940s

By the early 1940s, the prevailing medical theory was that brain dysfunction caused serious social and interpersonal problems. In terms of hyperactivity, severe cases were thought to be the result of brain injury, while less severe cases were blamed on poor parenting or 'overstimulation'. While research slowed during World War Two, by 1947 a new medical theory – Minimal Brain Damage – emerged that linked brain damage at birth with hyperactive behaviour.

The 1950s

These were boom years in the US for medicating psychological problems due to the belief that science could cure the world's ills. There were high hopes for the capabilities of drug use, and advertising campaigns by pharmaceutical companies took advantage of this mood. Overactive and impulsive behaviours were just one of many conditions increasingly treated with drugs, and it was in this decade that methylphenidate (Ritalin) first became available to families. This link between medication and behaviour had a big impact on medical research, with a renewed emphasis on amphetamines to treat mild as well as severe forms of hyperactivity. Reflecting on this development almost 20 years later, a leading US researcher in this area, Dr Maurice Laufer, claimed that the impact of his research continued to surprise him – he'd never intended all misbehaviour to be attributed to brain abnormalities, he said, nor had he expected amphetamines to replace non-biological treatments.

By the mid-1950s, scientists were using new brain-scanning equipment to find a biological cause of behaviour problems, but no sign of brain damage could be found. Given that no cause was found (despite improved technology) you'd have expected some serious debate about how valid the existing medical theory was. Yet the medical theory for behaviour problems persisted – although there was a change to the label. To accommodate the failure to pinpoint brain damage as a cause, the name of the disorder gradually changed from Minimal Brain Damage to Minimal Brain Dysfunction. This changed again in the late 1950s when a new label, Hyperkinesis, was coined to describe milder forms of hyperactivity.

The 1960s–1970s

By the 1960s and 1970s the promotion of drug treatment by pharmaceutical companies had made some impact. Health professionals and the public became increasingly aware of medical theories to explain hyperactive behaviours. With this came more debate about the issue, and by the early 1970s the Hyperkinesis label was under attack for being too vague. Research also appeared to discredit the theory that responding to amphetamines proved that children with hyperactive behaviour had different brains.

In response, another label, Hyperactivity, emerged to describe behaviours like impulsiveness, aggression, low self-esteem and hyperactive behaviour. Throughout the 1970s there was a growing acceptance that hyperactivity stemmed mainly from an inability to concentrate or to control impulses. This was an important step in the development of the ADHD label because it distinguished it from other problems like depression or lack of nutrients in the diet that could cause similar behaviours. The other important development at this time was a new emphasis on both impulsivity (a persistent inability to think before doing or saying something), and on inattention (an inability to concentrate on tasks or listen to instructions). This shift to include inattention made a big difference because it broadened the range of problems that could be considered for drug treatment – and meant that more children were suitable candidates for medication. However, this new theory was not without its critics, with some experts arguing that the Hyperactivity label didn't represent any real progress in research – instead, it was just a repackaging of old theories (resulting from a growing social acceptance of drugs to treat mental illness, as well as a wider philosophical shift to treat poor behaviour as a disease).

In this way the first serious questions about the social impact and cultural influences of the disorder began to be raised. Until the 1960s the condition was the subject of only medical research and scrutiny, and for this reason it sneaked beneath the radar of many social researchers. Further, the many label changes since the theory first emerged caused confusion and made it hard for social debate to keep up. So it's not surprising that few questions were asked about the social side of the condition.

The 1980s

The new developments of the late 1970s had significant professional support – especially when in 1980 the American Psychiatric Association made the term Attention Deficit Disorder (ADD) official by including it in its bible of psychiatric diagnoses, the *Diagnostic and Statistical Manual*. By 1987, the label had changed again to Attention Deficit/Hyperactivity Disorder (AD/HD) and Undifferentiated Attention Deficit Disorder (U-ADD). U-ADD referred to children whose problem was mainly inattention, rather than a mix of inattention and hyperactivity. All these changes just added to the confusion, and by the end of the 1980s it was not uncommon to hear authors, researchers and professionals using a dizzying range of labels, including Hyperactivity, ADD, ADD+H, ADD-H, U-ADD and AD/HD. Again, debate outside medical circles struggled to keep up.

The 1990s

It was in 1990 that Russell Barkley, now an internationally recognised expert on the medical theory of ADHD, released his book *Attention*

Deficit Hyperactivity Disorder: a handbook for diagnosis and treatment. In it, he argued that the disorder was a genetically inherited physical condition that limits a child's impulse control and progresses into developmental disorders of social control and attention. His book's clear explanations had an immediate impact, increasing awareness of the disorder in the US and Australasia.

Although ADHD had not been well known, was rarely diagnosed and scarcely treated with drugs through the 1980s, diagnosis and treatment grew dramatically in the early 1990s. By 1994, when the American Psychiatric Association endorsed the new label 'ADHD', it was well known both here and in the US. While doctors kept pace with these name changes because they were the ones creating them, other people like teachers, social workers and psychologists whose work also involved ADHD struggled to grasp the differences between the various medical theories and labels. This meant that different professionals were often using different labels for the same problem, making it difficult for different specialties to work together and analyse the medical theory.

During the late 1990s ADHD theories continued to develop, with Russell Barkley suggesting that ADHD might have more to do with impulse control and inattention and that – again – we might need a new label to better understand the disorder. Nevertheless, at the time of writing, the label remains the same, a pause which has enabled an opportunity for exploration of the social side of ADHD.

What's in a label?

All these medical theories have had an associated label and, consequently, understanding labels is an important part of understanding ADHD. Labels can be important – giving a problem a name makes it easier to communicate about possible solutions. In medicine, putting the right label on a problem – making a diagnosis – is essential for providing the best treatment.

The benefits

Labels can help in other ways. In the case of ADHD, if you're over-whelmed by your child's hyperactive, impulsive and often aggressive behaviour and go looking for a cause, the label can provide a name and explanation for what can be a bewildering situation. It can also give your problem credibility. Parents of children with ADHD, for instance – often battered by the scepticism and condemnation of other people – can explain their child's problems as a real condition backed up by the medical profession. When a child stigmatised by labels like 'uncontrollable' gets a new 'no fault' medical label, it helps lift the burden of guilt and families are reassured that their struggle has a real cause.

When a child stigmatised by labels like 'uncontrollable' gets a new 'no fault' medical label, it helps lift the burden of guilt and families are reassured that their struggle has a real cause

Labels can also provide a light at the end of the tunnel. Along with an explanation, the ADHD label brings a range of treatments – including stimulant drugs that usually have dramatic and immediate results. The label is also a way of separating the child from their behaviour. This can boost self-esteem because it allows a child or young person to build a new identity as a good child with problem behaviour or troubles at school, rather than just as a 'problem' or 'trouble' child.

You can use a label to get more help. When research confirms that a problem is real and significant and gives it a name, you're in a better position to ask governments and others to show more compassion and to provide better resources. Labels are often used to argue that it's inhumane to neglect a person who's struggling in a situation that science has shown is not their fault.

The drawbacks

But a label can also create problems. While it can help make sense of what's happening to someone, it can also become an expectation rather than an explanation. With ADHD there's the risk that labelling may stunt a child's potential. If the rest of the world sees the child only through the lens of an ADHD label and the child learns to define him- or herself as ADHD, then there's the risk of an 'I can't do that because I've got ADHD' attitude. The child may then only behave and grow within the limits of the label.

Labels can come to dominate a child's identity so that every difficulty he or she has can be blamed on ADHD even when it's not the cause. In this way the label can stop them finding ways of dealing with problems that may be unrelated to ADHD. It can also be used to excuse behaviour that has nothing to do with the disorder. Anyone who's a parent or works with children knows that, ADHD or not, they all try to get away with what they can, and there's always the risk that any label (whether it's asthma or ADHD) can be used to justify why they do – or don't do – something. For instance, if a child doesn't do his or her homework, does something vindictive rather than just impulsive, or forgets to bring a note for his or her parents home from school, there can be a temptation to 'blame his or her ADHD'.

Another danger with labels is that they can set people apart. As some disability researchers point out, using labels to highlight the fact that someone is different can get in the way of any attempts to promote inclusion and have them valued holistically. Labels like ADHD can also tell us something about our social attitudes. The school of thought that studied labels and society in the 1970s was called 'Labeling Theory.' It was built on the observation that people get edged out of mainstream society because they break the rules that other social groups create. This may seem blindingly obvious, but what this theory argues is that it's not your personal qualities that make you an outsider but rather the label other people stick on you. In the case of ADHD, this theory suggests that the cause of the problem might have as much to do with the power of society to make us see a young person as deficient, as it does with what young people actually do.

Social researcher Peter Conrad used 'Labeling Theory' to look at how hyperactivity evolved over time, and pointed out that medicine had come up with a medical way of controlling over-active behaviour – psychostimulant drugs – long before doctors developed a sophisticated medical theory. Conrad, the author of *Identifying Hyperactivity in Children: The Medicalisation of Deviant Behaviour,* believed that once science came up with a medical means of controlling behaviour, it was only a matter of time before someone came up with a medical label to warrant the use of the medical technology. His conclusion? That as long as medical technologies grew, so would new medical theories to justify the medical control of socially unacceptable behaviour. He presented the history of the hyperactivity label as one clear example of this.

The role of drug companies

From the history of ADHD presented above, it is tempting to do what ADHD critic Thomas Armstrong does – blame doctors, activists and pharmaceutical companies:

> 'Essentially, then, ADD appears to exist largely because of a
> unique coming together of the interests of frustrated
> activist parents, a highly developed psycho-
> pharmacological technology, a new cognitive research
> paradigm, a growth industry in new educational
> products, and a group of professionals (teachers, doctors
> and psychologists) eager to introduce them to each other.'

While I believe that blaming the growth of ADHD on drug compa-nies is misleading – neither should we ignore their contribution. As mentioned previously, there was in the 1950s and 1960s a strong belief in the ability of science and medicine to solve the world's problems. Drug companies aggressively promoted their products and many Western countries became eager consumers. In Australia, the 'Bex' era (which lasted into the 1970s) saw a broad cultural acceptance of that popular painkiller, which led to problems such as kidney damage. More recently, there has been a growth in the use of anti-depressant drugs for psychological and social problems – and some people argue that it's not surprising that the growth of Ritalin to treat ADHD in the US so closely followed the rising popularity of Prozac.

As consumers have increasingly come to believe that drugs can fix most problems, drug companies have grown rich and powerful. In the case of ADHD, drug companies have used this wealth and power to fund further research into medical theories and trials of drug treatments. While this isn't a bad thing, the downside is that drug companies only fund research that improves or protects their own position in the marketplace, and the limited funding from other sources for non-drug research only makes our understanding of ADHD even more unbalanced. If you only fund medical research, you only get medical results, medical theory and medical answers. This gives the impression that the only explanations for ADHD are medical ones – and this reinforces the use of drugs as well as influencing the scope of government policy.

Another way that drug companies have used their power is as a lobby group. Currently, Australian drug companies are negotiating to have slow-release Ritalin made available, which follows on from their recent success in having Ritalin listed on the Pharmaceutical Benefits Scheme. The slow-release version, which lasts around six hours, depending on the child, means children don't need to take medication at school. In addition, the power of drug companies to lobby policymakers shouldn't be underestimated. When I worked as a parliamentary advisor, representatives of international drug companies often contacted me to tell me of the latest developments to expand the availability of ADHD drugs on the Australian market.

There have also been claims that drug companies have influenced the growth in ADHD through direct funding of ADHD advocacy groups in the US. ADHD expert Dr Lawrence Diller alleges that in 1995 Ciba-Geigy (the makers of Ritalin) had contributed over US$900,000 to the leading American ADHD advocacy group, Children and Adults with Attention Deficit/ Hyperactivity Disorder (CHADD) – but CHADD hadn't revealed this donation to either its members or the general public. It's this support group that has driven much of the promotion of the medical theory of ADHD to parents and the public through videos, books and other resources. Claims such as these raise concern about the possible influence of drug companies, not only on a supposedly independent group, but also on the public that turns to such groups for information.

The mass media

If drug companies and activists are not alone in promoting the shift of ADHD from an obscure medical theory to a well-known phenomenon, then who else has been influential? One clear influence that continues to be important in the rise of ADHD is the media.

It was late in the afternoon, about midway through my interviews at Eastside High School, my second research site. Charlie was sitting at a desk paying close attention to what we were saying, while Steven sat at a larger table, swinging his legs. Charlie, who was almost 16 and tall for his age, saw himself very much as the young adult, while Steven, darker and with a brooding look, was two years younger. Steven had been diagnosed with ADHD for as long as he could remember, while Charlie's diagnosis was more recent.

When the conversation turned to some creative activities that we might do over the next few interviews, Steven came to life.

'Can we make a video about ADHD and send it to "A Current Affair" and show Ray Martin that he's crap?' he said, his legs swinging more vigorously.

'Yeah,' said Charlie chiming in. 'What I hate is people like on "A Current Affair" and shit like that … they talk about what ADHD is and everything but they don't have … they don't have any conception of what it's actually like.'

I asked how they would show what ADHD was like, but Charlie cut me off, saying that the media exploited only the most severe cases of ADHD. 'They should stop going for the ratings and take time out to actually explain what ADHD is, and show that not all cases are severe.'

I was taken aback by the passion and content of Charlie and Steven's comments. It had been just another casual afternoon chat about what activities we would do during the next few interviews. Then, out of nowhere, these two teenagers began venting their anger. While not always as heated as Charlie and Steven's response, concern about the way media ignores the voices of young people with ADHD (such as those included in this book) was a constant theme in my interviews with teenagers.

From a relatively obscure diagnosis, ADHD has burgeoned into a phenomenon in Australia and the US, a growth reflected not only in the increased number of ADHD diagnoses but also in the interest of the media. In the last decade, media reporting of ADHD has helped shape a popular interpretation of the disorder that's only loosely linked to medical theories and isn't always accurate. To be fair, media attention is often a sincere attempt to make the public aware of the plight of children with ADHD and their families – but it would be naïve to pretend that ADHD doesn't make sensational viewing.

As families in the US fought for recognition of the needs of children with ADHD through the early 1990s, the media was an obvious avenue for raising awareness. The media gave parents an opportunity not only to lobby for better resources and support but also to break down notions of poor parenting as the cause of ADHD.

Journalists saw a good story in the issue of using amphetamines to treat socially unacceptable behaviour, while parents, keen to make sure the issue wasn't lost in the controversy about drug treatment, willingly offered their stories. Given the dynamite combination of volatile behaviours and the medical use of an otherwise illicit drug, it's no surprise that the media quickly embraced ADHD. Soon, American television networks were screening current affairs stories on ADHD, and major news programs such as '20/20' and 'Good Morning America' were including reports on the disorder and the growing controversy over its cause and cure.

With increased media coverage, more parents became aware of ADHD and explored it as an option for their children. As more young people were tested, more were diagnosed and medication rates grew, thus creating another controversy – why was amphetamine use growing so rapidly? This drew other professional groups into public comment on this issue, and the media then had a range of conflicting views over the appropriateness of diagnostic practices and possible overdiagnosis. With each new media report on ADHD came more controversy, and soon a snowballing effect saw ADHD become a phenomenon of its own.

The history of the growth of ADHD through the mass media is an interesting one. Initial media reports in the US emphasised different brain activity among ADHD children and the use of psychostimulants as a miracle cure. As with medical research generally, the media's rush to be the first to report new findings, and the limited time they have to explain them, often means that flaws in a new study – or the fact that a study is very small or only preliminary – are glossed over. This is how many media health stories become oversimplified and send a distorted message. Yet once these findings become public, they take on a life of their own, and any reservations about the research are often overlooked.

A classic example of this was the media's reporting of Alan Zametkin's study (see Chapter 2), which found that some parts of the brains of parents of ADHD children used less of the brain's main fuel – glucose – suggesting that perhaps these areas of the brain worked less effectively. As ADHD is thought to be genetic, the assumption was that their children's brains would be the same. What wasn't so widely reported was that it was only a small preliminary study – and that it hasn't been backed up by any further research. But this trend to tell only half the story became typical of many media reports of ADHD.

Another crucial development in the media history of ADHD was a 1994 *Time* magazine article on the work of clinical researchers as well as the views of the growing number of ADHD support groups. It presented the view – popular among these groups – that ADHD was a biological reality. The article focused on the stories of individual children, and, in particular, the positive change that medication made in their lives. Most importantly, it repeated the misrepresentation of the Zametkin study to an even wider audience of readers outside the US.

With each new media report on ADHD came more controversy, and soon a snowballing effect saw ADHD become a phenomenon of its own

However, by the late 1990s attitudes toward ADHD in the media were shifting, a trend highlighted by a 1998 story – again in *Time* – which reported sensational stories of hyperactivity while also raising concerns over the growing numbers of children diagnosed with milder cases of ADHD. By pointing out that some parents (even those who were reasonably comfortable with their children's behaviour) felt pressured to medicate their children so their behaviour would conform, the story showed how the popular view of ADHD was changing. Reports like these only acted as a trigger to further media coverage, and it was only a matter of time before ADHD became a major topic of interest to the Australian news media.

Since the late Nineties, Australian commercial TV current affairs programs have regularly run stories on ADHD (predictably, not long after the start of each school term). The theme of these stories has usually been the use of different treatments for ADHD and the dramatic rise in drug use. Typically, they include footage of a mother screaming at her child as he runs wild within the house. After presenting parents as being at their wits' end, there's a brief report on how a drug (or new non-drug) treatment has changed their lives. None of these snippets are comprehensive, nor do any of them explore the claims in detail – but they do make riveting viewing.

More recently, ABC television has produced stories on ADHD as part of its 'Health Dimensions' current affairs program. These reports, and the 'Catalyst' program in particular, did include the growth in drug use, but tended to explore new treatments and research in more detail. Notably, in 2000 the ABC also ran the multi-award-winning drama series 'Kid in the Corner' from the UK's Channel Four, which told the story of eight-year-old Danny, who struggled with behavioural problems. His parents' jobs were suffering, their marriage was at breaking point and his sister was having problems. When his father cracks under the pressure, he assaults Danny and walks out, leaving his wife to cope on her own. It's then that an ADHD diagnosis emerges as a solution, but with it comes the controversy of drug treatment. This realistic and responsible exploration of ADHD issues was widely watched by both educators and families, and was highly influential in Australia.

Other examples from late 2004 include singer Natasha Bedingfield making reference to ADHD in her number one Australasian hit, 'These Words'; Bart Simpson continued life after being labelled by Principal Skinner in 'The Simpsons'; and the children's cartoon 'Hilltop Hospital' showed Harry Hedgehog going to the doctor for his ADHD. Such media presentations of ADHD are not lost on children with ADHD. The media is more than just a vehicle of news, advertising and entertainment – it is also one of the main means of generating and promoting popular culture.

Today's children are exposed to a lot of media and popular culture, and what they see and hear can influence their identity at a critical time in their development. If young people come to believe that life's meant to be the way the media presents it, this raises questions about how young people with ADHD come to see themselves. In my research, the impact of media portrayals of ADHD had a real influence on how the students saw themselves – but more about this in the next chapter.

There is little doubt about the effect the media has had on ADHD in the United States:

> *'The attention paid to ADD by the media since the early*
> *1990s has undoubtedly contributed to the boom in*
> *diagnosis and Ritalin use. News reports tend to exaggerate*
> *the positive findings of scientific studies while downplaying*
> *studies that demonstrate negative results. Journalists*
> *favour simple story lines with easily identifiable heroes and*
> *villains, good and evil sides, black and white answers.'*
>
> **Dr Lawrence Diller**

Over the last decade, the mass media has taken the previous promotional efforts of the pharmaceutical companies and lifted them another level to contribute to the growth of a popular understanding of the disorder. Even though this understanding is only loosely linked to the medical theory and isn't always accurate, it's still used by people to make sense of ADHD, to form opinions and to shape identities. It's another reason why we should ask more than medical questions about helping kids with ADHD.

ADHD *and the Net*

There are now very few of us that do not have access to the Internet either at home, work or school. As the Internet has grown, so too has the presence of ADHD on this medium. In mid-1997, when I typed the term 'ADHD' into various search engines as part of my research, the search engine Hotbot recorded 18,362, entries while Yahoo recorded 35 sites devoted to the topic. In mid-2003, when I repeated this search, Hotbot turned up 57,570 references and Yahoo found over 71 sites. A recent search of Google returned over 800,000 entries for 'ADHD', and this figure continues to grow.

The Internet has contributed hugely to the growth of the ADHD phenomenon. Not only has the amount of information on the disorder increased dramatically, ADHD (or 'ADD' as it's often called online) is one of the most common childhood disorders you'll read about on the Net. Online resources virtually burst at the seams while Internet chatrooms are constantly abuzz with ADHD support strategies and controversies. But the problem with much of the information available online is that it's not always credible, and it can be difficult for the average user to know how legitimate or accurate some of it is.

One of the strengths and challenges of the Internet is that anyone with a computer can contribute. This freedom is a strength when it comes to giving a voice to people who aren't often heard in debates about ADHD, but it's a challenge when it comes to providing accurate reporting of recent research into the disorder. Anyone can use the Net to promote their theory of cause and best treatment, from the well-meaning to the misleading.

When a parent gets on a site that talks about the lives and experiences of families of children with ADHD, he or she has their own life experience to help measure the legitimacy of a site's claims. However, when a site reports on scientific research results and possible cures, families in need rarely have the time or expertise to assess how valid these claims are. When you publish research in a peer-reviewed scientific journal it has to meet certain standards, but because there are no rules on the Internet it's easier to publish questionable research that wouldn't make the pages of a respected publication.

The result is an ADHD Internet phenomenon that has more to do with pseudo-science and popular opinion than credible research. Like the rest of the media's representation of ADHD, the ADHD we see on the Internet is often something that many scientists scarcely recognise.

It's not hard to trace how ADHD has integrated itself with the Internet. Searching on the web has a sense of personal discovery as well as a sense of individuality. For a person or family who feels misunderstood and persecuted by others, finding a solution on the Internet that seems to make sense can be a huge relief. The Internet is seen as a tool of revelation as well as a reassurance that ADHD is not their fault.

What the emergence of the Internet has done in the history of ADHD is to cap off a process that started with pharmaceutical companies and the media

The Internet also provides communities of common interest. At one time, communities sprang from people living closely together – now they evolve online as people search the Net until they find others of like mind. But the problem with too many like minds together is that you can end up with tunnel vision. Losing the tempering influence that comes from mixing with people who disagree with you and, instead, gaining the constant reaffirmation of the like-minded can create a false sense of reality. While many people use the Internet responsibly to create support networks, it can also attract those who feel alienated and misunderstood, encouraging an 'us and them' or a 'black and white' view of the world.

The Internet is also a very efficient way of spreading information rapidly, and one cannot underestimate how the Net has helped flood the world with information about ADHD from the home of ADHD and the Internet – the United States. Previous studies have shown how information about ADHD spread across Western countries as doctors trained in the US carried the message out. Now, with the Internet, these doctors no longer need to leave home to have a global impact. The growth of ADHD online may well be behind the recent interest in ADHD in the UK and Europe, where traditionally professionals have resisted ADHD.

There's also a sense of currency with the Internet. People prefer to research on the Net because it is the latest, most exciting and interactive. This is a reflection of the love of technology in Western culture – many people trust what they find on the Internet more than they do their own judgement or even that of health professionals. The idea exists that any information to do with computers has great credibility, a generalisation that echoes some assumptions we see with ADHD – namely, that if someone in a white lab coat endorses something (be they a doctor or a scientist) then it must be credible.

What the emergence of the Internet has done in the history of ADHD is to cap off a process that started with pharmaceutical companies and the media. It has further expanded public awareness of an obscure medical theory to the point where it has become a part of popular culture. The power of the Internet is that it feels more personal. It plays an important part in connecting those who live with ADHD and reassuring them that they're not alone in their struggle. It's also an important tool for raising public awareness of the difficulties families face and their need for support. Yet the same tool can also be used to promote money-making cures, misrepresent research findings and peddle myths. Like any technology, it is not in itself bad, but with no way to check the legitimacy of many of these claims, the danger of the Net is that it provides more scope for ideas to emerge that have little to do with the medical theory of ADHD.

Key points

- The evolution of ADHD has more to do with social and historical change than it does with refinements of the medical theory.
- Although science got the ADHD ball rolling, the media has made it something that the scientists scarcely recognise.
- Young people are influenced by the presence of ADHD in popular culture, and this needs to be considered in treatment.
- Labels like ADHD can be both useful and harmful, and can also be windows into the values of the society that applies the label.
- While the rapid change in labels has stunted non-medical debate about ADHD in the past, the recent stability of the label has enabled greater social consideration of ADHD.

4

Living with ADHD – teenagers' stories

'... this is the first year I have ever done like any work at all at school, I never used to do anything at all at primary school ... this is basically reception for me...'.

'So what is the thing that has changed to make this happen?' I probed.

'It's heaps hard. I can't do like ... look, I don't even know my times tables ...', Ben paused, exasperation in his voice. 'I never learnt anything in primary school ... 'cause I never used to do anything ... I had ADD but no-one knew what that was ...'

'So now you're trying to catch up?'

'Yeah, I'm still in reception here, man ...'

Ben, 13

A dolescence can be difficult enough for any young person. It's a time of real upheaval – not only are teenagers shifting away from parents to rely more on their peers, on popular culture and themselves to help shape their decisions, but they're also testing the boundaries. In a few short years they come to understand how they see themselves and are seen by their peers and others. Imagine how much more stressful adolescence is for teenagers who are already struggling with hyperactivity, impulsiveness, inattention, low self-esteem and poor social skills?

These changes make adolescence a rocky road for most teenagers with ADHD. Young people with ADHD – like all young people – need structure and support in their lives, but many adults make the mistake of dealing with conflict and risky behaviours with hard-line tactics (like enforcing strict guidelines, being more authoritarian and giving young people less of a say in decision making). This approach by parents or teachers is a recipe for disaster. Many teenagers find this alienating and condescending, and it does nothing to help develop the trusting relationships that are important for young people in these crucial years.

Support from home and school are crucial in helping adolescents with ADHD to reach their full potential. This support means being positive, patient and understanding while setting clear rules and boundaries. Adolescents with ADHD overwhelmingly want to behave and do well at school, even though it's not always obvious to others. They're very conscious of their poor behaviour, and although they feel that having a diagnosis of ADHD can be helpful in some ways, it can also bring a sense of shame. This is why emotional support is so essential to adolescent self-esteem and why it's important not to confuse a young person's worth with the way they behave – in other words, separate the person from the behaviour.

Despite all its challenges, one of the great things about adolescence is that it's also a time of growing self-awareness when young people develop the ability to put forward their own views, rather than deferring to the values of parents. It's exciting to watch them form a concept of the world and their place in it, as well as notions of justice and equality. This process of moving into the adult world makes adolescents very perceptive about many things that adults have stopped seeing or take for granted. It is this keen awareness among teens that makes them a great source of insight into ADHD, which can help the rest of us understand it. Yet what stands out to me is that, despite all the research about ADHD, it's often the voices of those who are closest to it – the young people and families who live with ADHD – that are the ones we hear the least. When we do hear them, they're often filtered through the opinions of experts.

This is a gap that I've tried to fill with my own research in Australia and the US, and by including comments and anecdotes from the conversations I've had with young people with ADHD and their families in this book. I have tried as best I can to let their own words speak and not over-edit or 'play expert' over their words. The resulting stories are perceptive and moving. If we want to understand the disorder better and do more to help, the people we should be listening to are the young people themselves.

So, to give a sense of what it's like living with ADHD, I've included in this book some stories and poems written with and by teenagers that give a rare insight into ADHD. Many of these stories came out of interviews I did with high school students, so one recurrent theme is what they think about how schools deal with ADHD and how things could be improved. They also talk passionately about the distress that comes from wanting to do your best, but having a disorder that gets in the way. The stories show how keenly aware these teenagers are about how their behaviour affects their families. There are many other themes, insights and concerns woven into the stories of the next few pages, and these I address through explanatory notes about key concepts.

These stories and poems are a clear statement by the teenagers in my research about how they see the world. It was them, not me, who created the following stories – two from groups of students in South Australia, and two from students in Nebraska, in the US. The poems were also produced in collaboration; but my role was more significant in these. Put together, they shed light on how students with ADHD see themselves, the disorder and the environment they try to function in.

Stories from the inside

'Red the Squirrel'

Red was an adventurous squirrel
Who used to love a surprise
He would greet it with a smile
and a glint in his shiny eyes.

But last week after he left his tree
He's so solemnly sure
he'll never leave it again
– not after what he saw.

He'd scampered down to follow
the kids that passed each day,
kicking up autumn leaves
as they skipped along the way.

He followed until they went inside a building
(much taller than his tree),
which he scampered all around
to discover what he could see.

At last he found a dark oak tree
like the one he knew
and clinging to it halfway up
he got a better view.

He saw kids and tables,
pictures and chairs,
but still he couldn't work out
what was going on in there.

Red had heard of these places before
he'd heard kids call them schools
but he didn't know what they did
except teach facts and rules.

Finally the kids came out
and Red hatched a cunning plan:
he'd befriend a likely looking youth
and get carried in by hand.

He spied a blond young man
who looked like he was in for fun,
so Red carefully bounced up to him
in a sort of cautious run.

Well the plan worked well
and before much time could pass
Red had been smuggled in
to his first mathematics class.

The boy sat down to take out his books
and Red's problems started about then
because schools you see are not designed
for the likes of our adventurous friend.

There was too much to do and see
for Red to stay in the student's pack
so as soon as he opened it to get his books
Red scampered up his back.

The other students gasped and giggled
but the teacher didn't seem to see –
he was facing the blackboard
writing something about probability.

The student told Red to stay still on a seat
because that was what you do in school
and to do it Red tried and tried
but it seemed more than he could do.

Red was naturally full of energy
and not suited to sitting still
and doing that for half an hour
was an impossible act of will.

So Red shuffled around
avoiding the teacher's glance
trying to explore this thing school
making the most of his chance.

But Red couldn't seem to learn anything
because the teacher just droned away,
and because he struggled to read or write
there seemed no point anyway.

So eventually when the teacher came
to escort him back outside
he was kind of glad it was over
and scampered home to hide.

Maybe Red could have liked school better
if he had learnt how to behave when young,
or maybe it just was the way he was,
so, once born, the deed was done.

Or maybe if the teacher hadn't droned on,
or had taught with squirrels in mind,
Red might have learnt more
and had a far less harrowing time.

Or maybe if schools were about something else
and taught for different sorts,
maybe then Red could've fitted in
or at least lasted until sport.

But now safe back in his tree Red knows
that school is not for him,
and when he sees the boy in the yellow school bus
he gives him a knowing grin.

Note: 'Red the Squirrel' is based on an interview with a teenager in Lincoln, Nebraska who described his difficulties at school and how he wished he was one of the squirrels he saw on the way to school each day.

Baldy's story

There was one thing Archibald Nehemiah was sure of – that no-one would ever call him a 'geek'.

Sometimes kids called him 'speedy boy' because he had to take medication every day, but he just ignored them and told them where to go. But a 'geek' was one thing he couldn't stand being called, and he made sure that anyone who did, didn't do it again.

Being called Archibald didn't help. Arch or Archie was even worse; man it pissed him off when teachers called him Archie.

So if someone gave him shit, nothing was more certain than that he gave more back. That was probably the reason he was starting a new school today.

He'd regretted beating the kid up for calling his mum a 'bitch', but when someone hassled his family, he saw red, and just had to beat the crap out of them. No-one, no-one gave him or his family shit.

Although this morning was his first at a new school, it was the middle of term, and the day started like most other days. His dad woke him up when he started his old motorcycle to go to work at 7.30 a.m. The bike sounded like someone dry-retching gravel at the top of their voice. His mum would be in the kitchen cleaning up, as he'd slowly crawl out of his bedroom, over piles of junk and toward the shower, his face screwed up and covered with lines from his pillow.

After his shower he would get dressed, and put on his cap. He didn't have to comb his hair because Archibald was nearly bald. It was how he got his nickname 'Baldy', but only his mates called him that. Baldy had a number one crop and that was why he always wore his red Chicago Bulls cap to school. Normally he would have put on at least some of his school uniform, but today he didn't have to; his new school didn't have a uniform.

The next step in his routine was to go to the outside dunny to sneak a smoke, watching for Mum, because she'd go apeshit if she caught him smoking. But he'd been smoking since he was ten, so after three years he wasn't going to give up. The dunny was in the middle of a backyard that was like most people's in their Housing Commission area. It had an old shed with a lot of dust, cobwebs and things half pulled apart, a clothesline on a bit of a tilt in a cracked bit of concrete, and couch grass that would look dead in summer and go wild with runners in winter. There was an old swing from when they were little that they didn't use any more, his brother's bike rusting in the sea air, and, of course, the dunny, which had just always been there.

Baldy liked his home – it was the only place he'd ever lived.

After his smoke Baldy would sneak inside while his mum was getting his brother ready (so she wouldn't smell the smoke on his clothes). He'd take his tablets, and grab something to eat so his dexies didn't give him stomach pains. Then he'd yell, 'Seeya Mum', and before she had time to answer he was on his bike and on his way to school.

Baldy was proud of his bike. It was a chrome Redline, given to him by his family last Christmas. He had to guard it carefully because he didn't want it stolen or trashed. It had tuffs on its wheels, trick nuts on its axles and hardly a scratch on it after a year. Baldy was always proud when he cruised on his bike, without a helmet or cap, his scalp bristling and glistening in the sun.

Normally Baldy would have met his mates in the Foodland carpark and walked to school with them, just before the bell, but today he had to ride in the opposite direction to his new school. As he rode, he thought about the people he used to go to school with.

There was Billy, his best mate, who was always tired and never did anything he didn't absolutely have to. Billy was tall, skinny and scruffy, and always looked like he needed a wash, even after a swim. He talked a bit slowly but wasn't stupid, and he was really good at making stuff. Like the recess time they made soap bombs to throw at smelly Kelly – so cool. The girls didn't like Billy much. They thought he was ugly, but Baldy liked him. They had fun on weekends and used to run amok together in class when they got bored, which was most of the time.

Baldy didn't eat much, but Billy was always hungry, and Baldy reckoned it was because he smoked too much dope and got the munchies. Baldy smiled to himself when he remembered Billy's plan to order pizza one day and bring it to Care Group – the daily student teacher meeting that they had each day. It didn't work because the pizza guy went to the front office, and Billy got into heaps of shit. Billy said afterwards that it didn't matter, because if they had got the pizza to the Care Group, they wouldn't have got any because Whitey would have eaten it all.

Billy and Baldy hated Whitey. He was big, fat and white. No-one knew his real name, except the teachers, but they all hated him. He was a geek – everything Baldy didn't want to be. Baldy was glad he didn't have to put up with him being a dickhead every lesson and sucking up to Ms Pinkerton in Care Group.

Ms Pinkerton was alright, she'd let you get away with stuff and have fun in lessons, and she was like Ms Black, who tried to understand ADHD and help. They were better than Mr Pain, he'd tell you one thing one minute and another the next. He'd come into class in a bad mood and take it out on you, and anyone he didn't like he'd yell at and say 'You, yes you! You got a "U".'

Baldy reckoned all teachers had favourites, but because Mr Pain's favourite was Whitey it was even worse.

Baldy was going to miss Billy, but at least he could still see him after school. He probably wouldn't miss the others.

Even though he had visited this new school before with his mum, as he rode through the gate and locked up his bike for the first time he still felt those butterflies you get in the stomach at a new school on the first day. Baldy had changed schools lots of times before, but he still got nervous, especially as he went to the front office and stood around like a loser, waiting for someone to meet him and take him to class.

His parents had told him this was a good school that tried hard to help kids who don't usually fit in easily, but Baldy wasn't convinced. He had heard it all before. He also reckoned most teachers didn't care or couldn't be bothered, and hardly any of them made school fun – most said that it costs too much .

Baldy was slinging his bag from one shoulder to another as a boy about his age came up with a teacher. The teacher said, 'Archibald, this is James – he's going to show you around.' James smiled at the teacher and said to Baldy, 'Follow me, I'll show you around.' That was the last thing he said to Baldy until they came to a room, and James said, 'This is your room', and then vanished. Baldy hated the sorts of kids teachers pick to show you around. You either get one who has their own friends and dumps you straight away, or you get a dud who takes weeks to get rid of so you can make real friends. Either way you end up fighting with them to find out how tough they are, or to show them you're not weak.

Baldy took a deep breath, opened the door to the classroom and went in. The first thing he noticed was that the room didn't look like a classroom. In the middle there was a big circular table shaped like a doughnut, with cords coming out of the centre and laptop computers plugged into them. There were a couple of kids sitting at the computers. The room also had beanbags, comfy-looking chairs, and posters and projects everywhere. It looked more like a classroom in primary school than in high school.

The next thing Baldy noticed was that there were hardly any people in the room. He'd just decided that there must have been heaps of kids away sick, when the teacher stood up from where she'd been sitting on the floor and came over.

'Hello, you must be Archibald,' she said with a big smile.

'And you must be a dickhead with a smile like that,' he thought, but he only said, 'Yeah.'

'Well, Archibald, I am Ms French, and this is your new class.'

Baldy had only seen scenes like this in crappy American movies.

She waited for a reply, and not getting one, moved on. 'Well, I'd best show you around.'

She showed him his locker, which had books, paper, pens and a new school bag in it for him. She showed him his chair, for what Ms French called 'group times', which was way better than the plastic ones he used to have to sit on that gave him backaches.

And then something happened that really amazed him. Ms

French said, 'And here's your laptop computer. Have you used a laptop before?'

Ms French didn't notice as the whites of Baldy's eyes showed, and his jaw dropped. 'My ... umm ... my laptop?' he stuttered.

'Yes,' she said. 'You can take it home with you if your parents agree to it. All our preparation work is done in the books I showed you before, but all our work to be assessed is done on your laptop and saved for me to mark. You can also use it to look at CD-ROMs and sometimes play games if you like.'

Baldy was speechless. *'Who's paying for this?'* he thought.

It was about then that the bell rang for the end of the first lesson, and Baldy moved over to pick up his bag for the next lesson. All the others in the room moved and sat down on the comfortable chairs, except the ones who were on the computers, who Ms French had to go and get.

They pleaded with her: 'Oh c'mon, Ms French, just a few more minutes. I just want to finish this level,' or 'Please, I've just got to get up to the next bit so I can use my cheat code, and then I'll save it.'

Ms French was firm, 'No, boys, you know the rules.'

Baldy put his bag down, and went and sat down with the nine or so other students. Already he could feel this was going to be a different day.

When Baldy got home, having had to carry his new bag and his old bag – but not the laptop – on his bike, his mum asked how his day went.

'It was really weird, Mum, like we stayed inside with the same teacher and stuff until the last two lessons ... and like at the end of each lesson, you get ten minutes' free time, like ... umm ... as a reward.'

'Oh yes,' his mum said. She probably wasn't listening.

'And, like, they said we could have a laptop. But you have to say okay, and we can play games on it, and can I have one?'

His mum was listening now. 'Well, Archibald, your father and

I have spoken about it, and you probably can, but we have to be sure you'll look after it.'

'I will. I can,' said Baldy speaking quickly.

'We'll see,' said his mum.

'And Mum,' said Baldy, moving on to the next topic, 'we got to do graffiti in art and there's like a graffiti wall that you can put your tag on and stuff, and they paint over it every week, unless it's a piece, cause then they leave it on longer...'

'Graffiti, I'm not sure about that ...' his mum said.

'And they let us draw while the teacher is talking,' he continued.

His mum stopped him. 'Well you seemed to have had fun, but did you learn anything today? What lessons did you have?'

'We, like, have the same lessons everyday, in the same order and that. After Group we had maths, and we made pyramid things and that, and worked out the volume and crap, but we got to talk at the end of class ... not that I knew anyone. And then we did computing and they were showing us the Internet ... and umm ... how to make websites ... and talked about viruses and stuff ... and then 'cause we were good we got to play games, and I played Virtual Ice Hockey, it's got cool fights ... and then we had recess ... which was a bit boring 'cause I didn't know anyone ...'

'Did you see Kerry? His mum told me he goes there,' she asked.

'I saw him, but I sorta hung around with the group on the oval. And after recess, which was short, we ... umm ... had English, where we got to act out the first half of a story and then write the ending ... and I used the spellcheck on the computer to get the words right. Then we just sat around and talked, which was a bit boring ... but like then we did science, that wasn't much different, but at the end we got to go out and play footy until lunch.'

His mum interrupted as he rambled on. 'How did lunch go then?'

'Lunch was really short, but I got to buy some stuff in the canteen – all they had was this health food stuff ... anyway I kept kicking the footy with the guys I kicked it with before. After lunch I did art ... like 'cause every term we swap and do tech studies, or home ec. or drama ... this term I do art ... and like at the end of the lesson I had finished my work and that, so I got to use the special soft lead pencils to draw something ... look I'll show ya.'

Baldy pulled out his carefully shaded and well-drawn picture of a Samurai warrior.

'I took all of last lesson to do it too,' said Baldy. ''Cause they haven't sorted my electives yet, Ms French let me stay in the room and finish it. I stuffed up the sword a bit, but she still said it was cool...'

'So did you learn anything today, Archibald?' Mum asked.

'Umm ... I got to use a computer ...'

'Well, see if you can have less fun and learn more tomorrow,' she said.

Suddenly it dawned on Baldy that Billy must be getting home about now, so he ran out, leaving the TV blaring and his mum shaking her head.

'The new school may be okay, but it's not as much fun as stuffing around with Billy,' he thought, jumping on his bike and heading toward Foodland. In a moment school was forgotten and wouldn't cross his mind again until his dad's motorbike woke him again tomorrow.

Notes on key issues

Family

One trigger for anger among the students was any sort of attack on their family. This was particularly true of students from single-parent families. Despite knowing how difficult they themselves make it for their families, young people with ADHD seem to be determined to make sure no-one else makes it any harder. These students were especially distressed when their ADHD was the reason for their parents or siblings being alienated.

Many students felt stressed both at school and at home because they were met by constant failure, despite wanting to do well. They felt guilty for the way they made life difficult for their families, and frustration because they could not seem to get things right. This stress continued even after a diagnosis and drug treatment.

Smoking

Social use of drugs, like smoking, was one way young people dealt with the stress of ADHD. However, this drug use wasn't widespread and varied according to the socioeconomic background of the students. Some smoked to help them calm down, while one used marijuana. Others, especially from upper middle-class areas, used caffeine and alcohol. But there was no suggestion that this social drug use came from any physical need caused by taking medication. If the students chose social drugs, it was either because of social expectations or because it helped them cope with stress.

Side effects of medication

One of the few side effects they reported from medication was occasional stomach pains. ADHD drugs can also suppress appetite and affect children's growth if they're used for long enough. Several students put their small stature down to long-term medication – some claimed to have been using drugs for more than five years, which is longer than recommended.

School computers

The students also agreed that the growing use of computers by teachers in schools is helpful. Computers provide interest, focus and help students complete tasks using a range of strategies, including non-linear thinking.

Firmness

Another strategy used by some teachers and appreciated by students was an emphasis on being firm but fair. As much as these teenagers resisted the limits placed on them, they still respected teachers who made the effort to set boundaries. Perhaps this contradiction reflects the students' own struggles with trying to regulate their behaviour and learning.

School procedures

They also pointed to a number of changes that schools and teachers can make to help them. Because the students found the organisational demands of high school very difficult, they appreciated being taught by only a small number of teachers and remaining in the same classroom. Another problem was coping with the change-over between lessons, particularly after lunch. They found it difficult to shift almost immediately from rowdy play to silent work. One change they suggested was a reduction in class sizes – students felt frustrated that the teacher never seemed to have time to help them, and this increased the chance that they would get distracted or bored.

Healthy eating

Students felt that eating the right food was important. Although diet is not a cause of ADHD, they recognised that it could contribute to behavioural problems. They felt schools could help by having canteens provide healthy foods with options that were low in sugar and preservatives.

Fred's story

It's 6.45 p.m. on another cold, dark June night in Adelaide. John and Fred are home trying to fill in the time before they go out clubbing. John's girlfriend Kate had arrived half an hour ago, already dressed up, but they hadn't moved from sitting in the lounge, watching television.

The house was typical of two single guys living out of home for the first time. It had its own smells and they never had to walk far to find clothes to wear. The lounge had plates and coffee cups in various parts of the room, possibly making their own way back to the sink. It was a small dim room, but with the bar heater going it was probably the warmest place in the old house. It had a television, three seats, a stereo and a CD rack made of a few bricks and two planks. The seats were all different, but they matched because of similar stains. It was probably better not to ask where the stains came from.

Fred was sitting on the large seat nearest the heater. If he stood up he wouldn't have been much taller than when he was sitting down, but he would still be fat. His body sort of rolled in and out with the seat, and in a bad light you had trouble telling which was Fred and which was the seat. He had his usual flannelette check shirt, army shorts and joggers on. His skin was pale and his hair short and cropped. People felt odd when Fred looked at them. Maybe it was because he had one green eye and one blue eye. Maybe it was just because he was weird.

John was lying on the sofa across from him. He was a lot skinnier than Fred, with brown hair, blue eyes and heaps of pimples. He was in his usual baggy no-label clothes that always seemed old about ten minutes after he started wearing them. John and Fred had been friends since Year Ten, and even though Fred had left school in the middle of that year, they had stayed in touch when all the others hadn't. John was hogging the lounge, making Kate cram into the tiny part of the seat that was left.

Kate and John hadn't been going out for long. They had met at a friend's party, got on with each other and it sort of developed from there. They hadn't really been out with anyone else before, so they thought they liked each other – but still weren't sure. Kate was in her first year at uni, training to be a teacher. John was unemployed, and Fred was doing night shifts stacking shelves at Coles.

Kate was about the same height as John. She had red hair, freckles and wore clothes from an op shop that were almost trendy. John's mum reckoned she was 'frumpy', whatever that meant. She was pretty loud when she talked and a bit moody; if she disliked someone they knew about it. She wasn't sure about John's taste in friends.

So there the three were sitting – Kate watching television, Fred telling weak jokes no-one was listening to, and John wondering how he could avoid buying Kate drinks so he could go out tomorrow night – when 'A Current Affair' started a segment on schools. It was about a kid who'd been picked on at school, and his parents complaining how schools should do more to help kids who are different.

This caught Fred and John's attention, and they started to talk about how school was crap when they went, and (forgetting Kate) wondering why anyone would want to be a teacher.

Kate, a bit put out, said: 'I betya that kid on TV is a little shit, I wouldn't want to be his teacher.'

'Probably like what we were, eh, John?' said Fred. 'Remember when I went in and changed all the passwords on the science lab computers. It took them ages to work it out, and there was no way I was going to 'fess up, but when Mr. Radkiwotiz found out, did he crack up at me. I got a week of binnies and an after-school for that.'

'Were you two good friends at school?' asked Kate, ignoring Fred.

'Nah', said John, 'Fred was too stuck up, thought he was too good for everyone else.'

'Piss off,' laughed Fred.

'No bullshit,' said John. 'Fred had only two people he'd have anything to do with, Tim and Joe. Tim because he would beat up on him, and Joe 'cause ... well I dunno why, he was just a square.'

Fred moved awkwardly in his chair. 'Joe was okay, just a bit spaced out, never talked much,' he said. 'But Tim, he was a dickhead ... Joe used to try and get me to like him but he was such a loser. He had that funny South African accent and went everywhere with his computer and never let anyone use it, and he wore clothes too small for him. He looked like John Howard ... a total geek.'

'So what was Fred like in Year Nine, John?' asked Kate teasingly.

'Dunno, we didn't really know each other. And he wasn't getting into trouble too much then.'

'No, I was still on my ADD medication then,' said Fred, deciding the conversation was better than 'Sale of the Century'.

'Have you got ADD?' asked Kate, genuinely interested.

'I did, I've kinda grown out of it.'

'I reckon Joe had ADD too, 'said John thoughtfully. 'He was smart but sometimes he was really vague. He sorta looked like the way Mr Burns in "The Simpsons" did when he walked out of the forest with big eyes.'

'Someone told me he was autistic,' said Fred, again trying to get a word in.

'No-one did anything about his ADD because no-one noticed. He only got in trouble with teachers when they asked him something and he was vaguing out and didn't answer,' said John, getting up and stepping on a dirty plate, which went 'clunk'.

'Yeah, but mine was different ADD,' said Fred to Kate. 'I was out of control as a kid, and then I got on medication and school was okay, but then I took myself off it 'cause I got worried about not eating and getting skinny and what it might do to me.'

'You've never been skinny,' stirred John.

Fred gave him the finger. 'After I came off my medication things got messy.'

'What do you mean?'' asked Kate.

'Well I got in more trouble for talking and eating in class, and not paying attention. John, remember how I'd get you into trouble too until we had that argument and the teacher made me sit down the front and treated me like I was some sort of freak? So I tried to sit up the back and she would make me sit down the front and make a fool of me, so I got angrier and angrier until one day when I lost it and just decked her.'

'You hit a teacher!' exclaimed Kate.

'I was really sorry straight after, but I got suspended. And I just said "Stuff it" to school.'

They were all silent for a while, each of them looking at a different part of the room.

'Yeah, but the problem was with the teacher. She was just hopeless.'

'When was this?' asked Kate.

'About the middle of Year Ten', said John.

'She was such a bitch, 'said Fred, 'Like I got on okay with a lot of other teachers, but she just cut me no slack. But once I hit her I knew I was gone.'

'It was a pity, 'cause we got a new principal not long after that and things got a bit better,' said John.

'What do you mean?' asked Kate.

'Well he got more special ed teachers to help students. People got help with organising themselves. Some were taught how to concentrate for longer and block out distractions. This principal got new equipment and resources so you could actually do something interesting. It used to be that you'd find something good, but the equipment was either stuffed or there weren't the right books in the library. Some of the teachers also made things more interesting by letting you work in groups or do projects you liked.'

'So the teachers changed too?'

'Well he made more classes that were smaller, and that made teachers less stressed and they had more time to help. He got rid of some of the crap teachers by having some minimum-standard thing.'

Kate looked thoughtful for a while, and Fred was trying to think of something funny to say but nothing would come to him.

Finally Kate said, 'We're getting trained about ADD at uni. They try to get us to leave things on the board longer, and understand that students can't help it. And they try to get us to concentrate on not interrupting the flow of the lesson.'

'Yeah, great,' said Fred. 'Still doesn't stop them getting angry and picking on kids.'

'Smaller classes made it better though,' said John, sensing the tension between Kate and Fred. 'And it meant teachers actually asked us more about what we wanted to do and stuff.'

'They still need training in personal skills. Some teachers were good, but most had little idea – they just did it for the money,' said Fred.

'You're just pissed off 'cause you got kicked out before it got better,' said John.

Fred ignored him. 'School's always sucked,' he said. 'Only way school would be any good is if students ran it.'

'But it'd be chaos,' said John. 'School has to stay as it is. You go there to get a job, that's all.'

'Done you a lot of good,' said Fred. 'I leave at Year Ten and get a job, and you go to Year Twelve and are on the dole.'

'Yeah, a job – as a night filler,' snapped John.

'Schools are stuffed,' said Fred, sulking.

'So what should they be like?' asked Kate.

'Like TAFE, with lecturers not teachers, and you can choose your subjects and you don't have to be there if you don't want. I had heaps of trouble at school, but I don't at TAFE. I don't get stuck with the same crappy teacher.'

'But there's not enough money to fix it, so everyone has to work harder. It's not the school's fault,' she said.

Just then, there was a knock on the door. It was Steve, telling them it was time to get going to the club. The conversation stopped there with the interruption, and Fred got changed and they were off. The lights were off but the heater and television stayed on ...

Notes on key issues

Priorities

Diet and size was an important issue for the students, as it is with most teenagers. Interestingly, while there was some stigma that went with having ADHD and taking medication, it was still preferable to being fat. One of the comments made frequently by the students was that their ADHD was more important to their parents and teachers than to them.

Image

Far more important to their sense of self was their ability to make friends and the kind of image they presented to others. ADHD only became a problem when it meant that they had no friends or appeared weird. Image was important in both the low-income and the middle-class school – though the images were different. While the students with ADHD in the low-income class school tended to emphasise tough and resistant behaviour, those from the upper middle-class school tended to emphasise dress and appearance. In this way, the students were not so different from most other students in these schools.

Where there was an important difference between the schools was the degree of stigma linked to using medication. In the low-income school there was some element of being 'cool' or 'tough' taking amphetamines. But in the middle-class school, students tried to keep their diagnosis and treatment secret, as did the school administration.

Medication

The students explained that medication enabled them to make choices. It did not automatically make them behave well or learn, but it did slow them down and enable them to think before they acted.

All the students saw a central role for drugs in the treatment of ADHD. This said, none of them wanted to stay on medication any longer than necessary, and they often talked about growing out of ADHD.

'Growing out of ADHD'

'Growing out of ADHD' was how the students described their reduced need for drugs as they grew older. Some explained that it was because they were learning how to behave better, while others believed it was because the parts of their brain that had been underdeveloped were maturing. Some didn't know why it was happening, but found they only needed medication for times of stress, like exams. Others found life without medication very difficult, and stood staunchly by their need for the label and access to medication. For many, growing out of ADHD provided the opportunity to find a new adult identity and question a label that meant more to their parents than to them. The attention of teenage students increasingly turns to social interactions and academic performance, making ADHD relevant only if it impedes these things.

Singling out

Students were upset by ADHD if it was used as an excuse to single them out in front of others. This can often result in violent outbursts of aggression and frustration – but often followed by real remorse after losing control.

Coping with the demands of school

These students want to do well at school and be liked by teachers and other students, but sometimes they feel that the demands on them outstrip their capacity to deal with those demands. This becomes more of a problem in secondary school as academic pressure increases. But the students had such good ideas for how school could help them cope better with these demands – many could be classed as good teaching practice for all teachers. These included:

* building up student self-esteem;
* making instructions clear and giving slower students time to copy things down;
* reinforcing learning points in visual and verbal forms;
* breaking tasks down into small steps;
* working in groups;
* having classes which alternated tasks that required concentration and tasks which allowed interaction; and
* placing greater emphasis on negotiation between teacher and student in the classroom.

Students were critical of how few teachers adopted these strategies. While they recognised that larger classes and poor resources made it difficult, they expected all teachers to use sound teaching practice.

Teacher quality

The students believed most people became teachers because they couldn't get a better job. The students also claimed that many teachers were poorly trained and had little idea about ADHD.

Billy's story

Billy lived in one of many towns named Springfield in America's Midwest. He was tall and slim for a nine-year-old, so he referred to himself as nine-and-a-half. Billy had cropped blond hair, blue eyes and was smart for his age … so smart, in fact, that he was two years advanced and went to middle school rather than grade school.

Billy lived with his dad, his sister George, his brother Bob, and little sister Junior (his mother had died when he was five). Bill's dad's name was Bob. Since he lost his old job as a salesman he had worked at a factory, often with double shifts, to try and support the family. George was 13, and while her dad was at work she took care of the others, especially Junior, who was three.

Their house was on the outskirts of town, not far from a creek which they liked exploring with their dog, Max. Often Bob would be out riding his bike while George was looking after Junior. Billy preferred to stay at home and read. He wished he had a computer. At school he spent a lot of time on the computers, but his family couldn't afford one. He had a lot of micro machines, and spent a lot of time playing with them. They were always spread around his room in the aftermath of the last battle. As a result, he didn't get much time to clean his room or do his homework, or any of the other boring jobs the kids were supposed to do. Often it ended up that the house was messy, and his dad would have to clean up, and he'd yell at George for not making them do it.

There was a lot of yelling at their house. When something went wrong, or someone said something without thinking, things were tense and George and his dad would get mad. Billy kinda felt it was his fault a lot of the time, because often he'd say or do things without thinking, and his dad would lose patience with him and yell something like, 'HEY STOP IT!' or 'HOW MANY TIMES …?' His dad had never hit any of them. Billy thought his dad was strict but fair. But often things weren't Billy's fault because the reason he did things without thinking was because he had ADHD.

Anyway, this story starts one autumn at Popstick Middle School in Springfield. George and Bob had been at the school for some time but Billy was only new, and some kids had started picking on him. The worst kid was John. He was bigger than Billy because he was two years older. But John wasn't as smart, and he resented that. John would ask Billy to help him cheat, or ask him for money, but Billy would say 'no', and then John would pick on him or tease him. This had been going on for weeks, but Billy had managed to be patient and put up with it because he did not want to get in trouble.

Billy's brother Bob knew what was going on, but he didn't want to do anything about it because he didn't want to risk his popularity. Bob was bigger than John, had short hair and brown eyes, and could have helped Billy, but he thought half the problem was because Billy had been messing around or brought it on himself. When the others called Billy a geek he sort of understood why they did it. To be honest, Bob was a bit jealous of Billy's intelligence. But Bob had more friends because he didn't annoy people all the time, like Billy did … so he wasn't going to risk his friends just because Billy was getting what was coming to him.

George didn't know about the trouble with John – well not until the famous lunchtime …

John had been picking on Billy for a few weeks now, starting off saying small annoying things and slowly moving towards bullying. Finally, one lunchtime, John tried to push Billy down the stairs and Billy just lost it. His face went all red and tears came in his eyes and he started yelling at John and hitting him, and didn't stop until a teacher came and broke them up. John tried to fight back but Billy threw himself at him so wildly that he had no chance.

Not long afterwards, the two of them were sitting outside the principal's office, both looking sullen and hurt. John was a little scared of Billy because he thought he was crazy, and Billy felt guilty about losing control.

When they spoke to the principal they both said it was the other person's fault. But somehow it seemed that Billy got into more trouble; maybe it was because the other kids described him beating up John.

Anyway, when Billy's dad came home he was still angry about the phone call he got from the school that day while he was at work. He was so angry he didn't wait for excuses, he sent Billy straight to his room. The principal had asked Billy's father to come and see him. Billy's dad had to find time to do this between his double shifts, and he was angry because he'd thought these problems were over now that Billy was in a new school. The last school had said that Billy's anger was due to being held back and being bored, so he'd hoped that getting him into a middle school would fix it. His dad knew Billy had ADHD and that it made things hard for him, but sometimes he just got sick of having to deal with problem after problem with Billy … while still having to bring up three other kids.

Billy had been sitting in his room for about an hour when there was a gentle knock on his door. It was Junior. Billy let Junior in and she sat on his bed and asked: 'Why're you here Billy?'

'I don't know, I don't remember,' he said, not wanting to talk about it.

'Why don't you remember?'

'Because I forget things, because I got ADHD,' he said as an excuse.

'What's that?'

Billy, being the smart kid that he was, went into a technical explanation talking about chemical imbalances, chromosomes, genes and medication, none of which Junior understood.

After listening patiently she asked, 'Do I get it too?'

'Maybe,' he said. 'You might because it's inherited ... you have to go to the doctor and they test you for three days and then they tell you, and if you do they give you tablets.'

'I don't want it,' she said. 'It makes Dad mad.'

Billy didn't say anything. He didn't like being reminded.

Having finished her conversation, Junior trotted out of the room and decided to go and check downstairs for Bob. Bob had just got home and was doing his homework in front of the television. Dad was still calming down in the kitchen with George.

'You got ADHD?' Junior asked Bob.

'What?'

'I don't want ADHD – it makes Dad mad.'

'You haven't got it,' said Bob. 'It's just Billy's excuse for being a screwball ... he gets all the attention and we suffer. I get sick of Dad being angry and all the bickering and fighting.'

Junior plopped herself down next to Bob and started watching TV with him. Meanwhile Billy's dad was in the kitchen complaining to George. 'It wasn't just the fighting,' he said. 'He's been disrupting his classes, rude to the teachers and destructive to things ... I'm sick of it ... this school was supposed to fix it.'

George knew better than to say anything.

'I know he should be on medication,' he went on. 'But we can't afford it ... not since I started working in the factory. I don't have the money and the insurance doesn't subsidise it enough. If we buy medication for him then the rest of us suffer.'

Billy's dad kept talking. 'The principal wants to know about his diet and his home life, as if it was our fault. If the school was looking after him properly we wouldn't be having this problem. I know Billy knows what he's doing, and has no excuses, but the school has to do something to help … besides just ringing up and complaining.'

'What are schools going to do?' asked George wearily.

'I don't know … maybe give him more homework, or some sort of counsellor support, or extend him somehow…'

Billy's dad didn't have the answers, he just needed to talk.

A couple of days later, when Billy's dad saw the principal, he suggested some of these things. The principal didn't say it, but he seemed to think that Billy's dad was using ADHD as an excuse. He said that Billy's concentration, or intelligence or learning wasn't the problem; it was his social skills and his behaviour toward other students and teachers. In the end, it seemed to Billy's dad that the principal was saying that they could help with learning but not with these other problems. The principal said the school would try a few things, but Billy had to improve his attitude.

Of course Billy's dad gave him a stern talking-to when he got home, taking away some privileges for a while. To Billy's credit, he tried really hard … but the school didn't really do much. They gave him a book where he got a sticker for every day of good behaviour, but Billy hated it because he thought it was condescending and treated him like a baby. He put up with it though because he didn't want to get in trouble again … when he got in trouble he'd always really regret it after when he had calmed down.

The school also gave him a homework book, which Billy's dad and his teachers were supposed to sign. It was meant to show he was getting special homework and that Billy was doing it, but after a while the teachers forgot to sign it and Billy's dad was too busy to notice.

So things didn't really change. Their house would blow up occasionally, Billy's dad couldn't afford medication, and every now and then Billy would blow up at school, and get in trouble. Billy didn't have any friends, and he hated school.

It was a pity that school went so badly for Billy because he was a really smart kid, and if it wasn't for his troubles he could have gone to college ... but Billy never reached his potential.

Notes on key issues

The 'poor parenting' myth
One myth about ADHD is that it's caused by poor parenting. Students had mixed feelings about this. They felt it was unfair to blame their parents, and although they acknowledged that parenting skills varied, they all stressed that poor parenting wasn't an issue in their situation. It was interesting to discover that the students also questioned the reality of the media version of ADHD they saw on TV – they felt many cases were so extreme that they must be either misdiagnosed or sensationalised.

Not their fault
ADHD was not seen as the fault of children themselves, despite the fact that the media sometimes implied this. In the students' minds, ADHD was a diagnosis of a real condition, although they also believed misdiagnosis could also happen. But as the only way to recruit students in the study was through records of diagnosis and drug treatment, it's not surprising that they all felt this way – to access drug treatment, they need to accept the label.

Not fully informed
Despite their acceptance of ADHD, few students knew what the initials stood for or what was meant to cause the disorder. Most explained that it was to do with their brain not working in the same way as other young people's, and that medication fixed the imbalance. What was much clearer in their minds was that it was inherited genetically.

Needs beyond literacy and numeracy
The place where ADHD caused the most trouble was school. Many explained that it was because of difficulties at school that their parents had had them assessed for ADHD. Part of this problem seems to be that the Federal Government has shifted the focus of learning support for students with difficulties to more support with literacy and numeracy. While this isn't a bad thing, it ignores the fact that many students, including those with ADHD, need help with other skills that help them learn. These skills include learning to listen while a teacher gives instructions, learning to sit still, and learning to work in a group without distracting either themselves or others. Without these skills it's difficult to learn anything. They also need the social skills to help them form positive relationships with others, including teachers and peers. In order to learn, children need to feel safe enough to fail – but if they feel alienated or have a tense relationship with their teacher and peers, this is difficult. Children need to feel safe with their teacher.

What teens say about ADHD

As these stories show, ADHD is more than just a medical diagnosis; it becomes part of an identity given to children by adults. The ADHD label and the drug treatment that goes with it come under new scrutiny as adolescents try to decide who they're going to be in the future. While few of the teenagers in my study regretted having been diagnosed with ADHD, most were concerned about the stigma of drug use and tried going off their medication at times. It's how well they manage in this period of testing life without drugs that's vital to their successful development of a non-ADHD adult identity.

In my research, I conducted over 100 hours of interviews with a dozen teens with ADHD. This, in addition to my many years as a teacher and youth worker, has seen one common theme: drugs enable a choice, they do not provide a solution. In my experience, teenagers with ADHD agree that drugs don't make kids learn or behave better; it just helps them choose.

This said, rarely were students aware of treatment other than drugs. Partly, this was due to their separation of ADHD from the rest of their life: they saw ADHD as a medical condition to be treated and did not link other problems with learning, organisation and building friendships to the disorder. This meant that if they did get other help for these problems they didn't see it as part of their ADHD treatment. But mostly, the lack of awareness of multi-modal treatment among both parents and students was because medication dominated their thinking about ADHD.

Teenagers in my research often also mention the stigma associated with taking drugs, but said that it wasn't as great as the stigma associated with their unacceptable behaviour. They frequently described the label and treatment as more important to their parents than it was to them. They did not see it as a label that tainted all parts of their life.

Teenage students with ADHD feel very guilty about their behaviour and the problems it causes for their family. This can express itself as protectiveness for their parents and siblings, which can act as a trigger to violent outbursts. Students living with ADHD feel a great deal of stress, and some use recreational drugs to help them relax. This drug use doesn't come from any physical addiction from using stimulants – but rather for the same reasons other adolescents try drugs, such as to help them relax and feel better or to be accepted.

In my experience, the consensus among teenagers with ADHD is that school is not cut out for them and they are not cut out for school. They earnestly want to do well, but accept that they won't fit in at school and don't expect things to change because it would take too much funding. They respect teachers who operate within the system in a firm but fair manner, but hate those who show little or no compassion for or flexibility with ADHD. What the students want is for teachers and schools to recognise that they are not stupid – they just learn differently.

> **Most children with ADHD don't fail because they don't understand schoolwork; they fail because schools do not understand how *they* work**

Students described school interventions as condescending. Often attempts to help them presumed that a lack of intelligence or skills, rather than difficulty with self-control and attention were behind the problem. A clear theme that came out of my interviews (and that runs through some of these stories) is that treatment can be thwarted by social influences. These can include problems with sitting still and concentrating, anger, conflict, learning, maintaining friendships, fights, and arguing with parents/teachers … the list is long.

Social and environmental influences are powerful at all times, and can become a barrier if they encourage a young person to set aside or give up on learning the skills they need to function as an adult in society. Examples of such skills at risk with ADHD include being able to:

- pick up on social cues;
- articulate feelings and concerns;
- build relationships with loved ones and peers;
- respond appropriately to the expectations of teachers and those in authority;
- resolve conflict;
- problem-solve;
- find legitimate outlets for energy/activity;
- advocate for themselves and others;
- respond to expectations in the community about ADHD; and
- participate in a democratic society as active citizens.

Unless possible social barriers to otherwise successful treatments are considered, these treatments may not help as much as they should. This is particularly relevant to schools. The message from the students was that most children with ADHD don't fail because they don't understand schoolwork; they fail because schools do not understand how *they* work. In particular, secondary school students found some remedial strategies frustrating (for example, the various literacy and numeracy programs that are currently available) and felt like they were being sent back to primary school. This in itself made students feel resentful.

At worst, students are put in a class of students of all ages with a similar problem and given a booklet to take them through the steps thought to have been missed in previous learning. A little better is when one-on-one support with a volunteer follows a similar process through pre-set packages to redress a problem by re-teaching it in a more detailed way. The use of some organisational and monitoring systems (such as a card signed each lesson by teacher and then parent) was seen to be demeaning. Also, short-term rewards and token economies in classrooms were seen as condescending when used only with them and not the rest of the class. Fortunately, these methods are becoming less common. If interventions for ADHD are to work, we must take account of the identity issues and social influences that are so important in the early teens.

The stories of teenagers with ADHD also show that growing out of ADHD depends on having the skills to survive at high school. If students learn the skills to negotiate the greater academic, organisational and social demands without using ADHD drugs, then they say that they have grown out of ADHD. Those who haven't learned these skills, tend to make ADHD part of their identity as a young adult. In this way, growing out – or not growing out – of ADHD can play a role in how young people form their identity.

One of the most important influences on how these teenagers see themselves – and are seen by others – is television, and they don't like what they see. Much of the anger they felt stemmed from not liking how they are represented. This is why building self-esteem is such an important strategy in helping teenagers with ADHD.

Adapting the label

'At first my parents weren't sure because they had been longtime non-believers in the fact that ADHD existed. Before that, all they saw was the stuff you see on the news and that, kids like beating up their parents, smashing houses up and that. And they'd just think that was just problem children ... and even I still have a lot of problems ... but not anywhere as big as someone who smashes up things or wrecks the house. But most people don't know that 'cause they think it's just another name for problem kids.'

Daniel, 13 years

'ADHD is sometimes, I think, overplayed, you know, in the media. They seem like they play the fact that some people

are misdiagnosed. They say that like everybody is … or this
could happen to you, you know what I'm saying? They
always try that card and they also stereotype, but it doesn't
really matter, it doesn't really mean anything if they do.'

John, 15 years

It is my observation that many teenagers create their own label
of 'mild ADHD'. This is because they don't want to be associated
with portrayals of ADHD in the media, but still feel a need for
some way of explaining their difficulties and getting support.

**Mild ADHD is an example
of how people who feel
powerless can empower
themselves by redefining
the label that other people
have put on them**

They felt the pressure to define
themselves as an 'ADHD kid' or a
'problem child' but knew there was
more to them than just one label. Although they didn't want to give up
the ADHD label entirely because it
could help them explain themselves
to others, they didn't want all the negative baggage that came
with it either. Their answer was to create a new, less stigmatising
label that could be included as part of their identity.

Like the children who use ADHD to try and avoid the consequences of their behaviour, this is another way in which students use the label for their own purposes. The stories of
teenagers with mild ADHD show that it's a mistake to assume
that they will just accept labels and identities. Rather, mild
ADHD is an example of how people who feel powerless can
empower themselves by either resisting or redefining the label
that other people have put on them.

It's not surprising that the recurring themes in teenagers' stories about ADHD include self-esteem and identity. If there's a challenge for these students, it's not so much living with the ADHD
identity as the lack of other legitimate or positive youth identities. Often the only identities that adolescents are presented
with are that of 'high achiever' or 'delinquent', and if you are

neither then you are expected to disappear. Young people with ADHD find disappearing hard to do, and their experiences highlight an important limitation in how youth identity is understood in Australia.

As Natasha Stott Despoja, the former Australian Democrats' leader, explains:

> *'Young people are a heterogeneous group – they are not a generic group, they do not have the same voice, the same views, the same mind. But with the media so often presenting young people as either overachievers or layabouts, gold medal winners or teenage criminals, governments and the Australian public often forget this diversity. Sometimes it seems that between these two extremes, there's a lack of legitimate identities available to young people.'*

Drawing attention to yourself because you're different puts any young person in a difficult position. But for someone wearing the ADHD label, it can be even more difficult. Through popular opinion and the media, the public is often encouraged to see these children as dangerous. Yet my experience of working with these young people is overwhelmingly the opposite. Their stories show that many will opt to identify themselves as mildly disordered rather than difficult, delinquent or disabled. If there's one telling phrase that came from my interviews with these students, it was that they were all keen to tell me they 'only had mild ADHD'.

'I only have mild ADHD'

He only has the mild form of ADD
he's not the hypo sort,
he's not a psycho like on TV
he just needs more school support.

But people say he would bounce off walls
and break out in violent fits.
People would see he's been to seven schools
and drove teachers out of their wits.

Yet some have seen the child within
the one with the engaging smile,
and some have seen he can start again
or at least succeed once in a while.

And could it be that while few respond without fear or favour,
he's just trying to survive saying 'It's only mild ADD behaviour'?

Note: 'I only have mild ADHD' was inspired by several months of interviews with students at an Adelaide public secondary school and written with the assistance of students with ADHD.

Key points

- The process of moving from childhood to adulthood makes teenagers keenly aware of their place in the world around them.
- Despite the views of teenagers being an important resource, we rarely ask them about ADHD, relying instead on the 'experts'.
- The stories of young people with ADHD show a complex mix of opportunities, obstacles, influences and identities.
- If there's one telling phrase that came from my interviews with these students, it was that they were all keen to tell me they 'only had mild ADHD'.
- Growing out of ADHD relies not only on learning the skills to survive high school, but also on building a legitimate non-ADHD identity.

5

Can boys be boys?

'Mum's been through heaps lately, like she almost had a nervous breakdown and that kind of stuff ... I thought it was my fault kinda thing, 'cause like my sister, she has ADHD but she doesn't get into much trouble 'cause girls don't get it as bad, it's the things I do that make Mum stress and that.'

Leon, 14 years, who has ADHD

Why do boys show more severe signs of hyperactivity? And why are more boys diagnosed with ADHD than girls? Generally, boys are four to nine times more likely than girls to be diagnosed with ADHD and treated with drugs, a statistic confirmed by Australian research. In this chapter, we will consider some of the reasons why this is the case.

Boys and ADHD

US research has shown that boys are not only more likely to be diagnosed with ADHD, but also that 50 percent of these boys lack the support they need to develop the kind of social skills that we all need to get on with other people. Similar research in Australia has shown that many young people with social skill needs fall through the policy support cracks. They find it hard to express their feelings, which build up and eventually burst out in anger or violence. Many lack the social antennae to detect subtle messages that tell us not to go too far. On a practical level, many annoy people, start fights and find it hard to keep friends. They constantly push the boundaries. It is not a happy picture. So why is this scene much more common for boys than for girls?

One argument is that ADHD is just part of the bigger challenge we're having with boys generally. Rates of depression and suicide among young males are disturbing. Education experts say more boys are struggling with literacy and schooling, while social scientists warn of growing violence, aggression and delinquency among young men. Others point to a confused sense of male identity, because male role models are not as clear as they once were. Many would say that the decline of the traditional Australian ideal of Anzacs, pioneers, jackeroos and tough sporting heroes has been healthy, with the resulting growth in the model of the Sensitive New Age Guy who can talk about feelings. Yet this is a situation still in flux, and many men and boys remain caught between conflicting ideals of masculinity. Teenage boys can find these mixed messages particularly challenging, and if you are prone to being impulsive and active you are increasingly being seen as a problem. Many people also

Many people wonder if ADHD is thriving because boys are having difficulty adjusting to a world that's changed so dramatically in the last 30 years

wonder if ADHD is thriving because boys are having difficulty adjusting to a world that's changed so dramatically in the last 30 years. Even a generation ago there was time and space for rougher and more adventurous play, but now the space for boys to be boys is not what it was.

A changed world

When I talk with my parents about growing up in the Adelaide Hills in South Australia, they reveal a world very different to today. They talk about a post-War time when people worked together to rebuild in communities of trust and cooperation. People would leave their homes unlocked and go away for days, children would roam the streets and fields (only coming home when it was dark), with parents confident that their children were known and safe. My parents tell of the shock of the John F. Kennedy assassination, the belief that murders only occurred in the US, and then their dismay as murders were reported in Sydney, Melbourne and then Adelaide. They recall the disappearance of the three young Beaumont children from an Adelaide football match in the late Sixties and how the attitudes of parents started to change. Doors were locked and children were kept closer. In a matter of 20 years, the world of adventure, energy and exploration of our children was significantly curtailed – we've seen a narrowing down of possibilities for our boys and a world with less room to be active and adventurous.

As a boy, I spent my formative years from five to fifteen in regional South Australia. I too had a taste of the world described by my parents. I remember building forts buried under dirt and tin, disappearing for hours on end and riding roughshod around the town and paddocks. My mother tells of her fear when we returned to the city in the mid-Eighties and how hard it was to adjust to the suburbs after country life. Now, twenty years on, many parents are too afraid to let their kids go to the local shops alone, and out-of-school sport is considered one of the few remaining safe activities (although this is proving increasingly costly). For these reasons, you are now more likely to find a boy playing alone on a Playstation than in a playground.

We also need to think about ways to open up and manage opportunities for boys to be active. For example, in my home city of Adelaide, I know many teenage boys who regularly go downhill bike riding in the nearby foothills. But this activity is constantly under threat because of tight council regulations, concerns about environmental damage and community fears that any group of teenage boys together must be trouble. Attempts to provide designated tracks continue to be thwarted, and it is ever harder for these boys to get out and let off steam. This is but one example of the few opportunities left for boys to be boys that we as a society curtail, but could be supporting. So, growing urbanisation and the reality of the increased density of city living may be another factor in the shrinking of opportunities for boys to be boys.

Further, as the space available for our boys has changed, so have our expectations of what's acceptable behaviour for boys. When it comes to dealing with relationship problems, schools now provide training to encourage boys to take a more traditionally feminine approach and talk through the issues. This is not necessarily a bad thing, but when their mates – and some adults – still reinforce that a quick punch-up outside sorts things out (so they can become best mates again), there are confusing messages. These contradictions create a tangled web of expectations for any boy trying to please parent, teacher and peer. And if you happen to be a boy who doesn't think things through before he acts, doesn't pick up subtle social cues, and expresses himself physically, it'll be so much harder.

A time-poor society

In addition, other social changes are not helping. Longer working hours and more families with two working adults means parents have less time to supervise free play, and their children are likely to spend more of their play time in an after-school or vacation care centre. At a time when it may no longer be safe to just let boys go and explore, and when it takes more effort from parents to find spaces for boys to be boys, we find that parents have less time to spare.

This lack of time also impacts on the exposure to positive role models of both sexes; and the modelling of respectful relationships between couples cannot be underestimated. If a boy is to learn how to act towards someone of the same or the opposite sex, there is no more powerful example than spending time with his father as a model. Yet the demands of an Australia that is among the most overworked nations in the world makes it hard for parents to play and even harder for fathers to be there. And I am sure that New Zealand is experiencing similar pressures. Some families have decided that parenting is to be a shared career, but in many professions and for stretched incomes this is often not an option. In a less-than-ideal situation, many boys will get by, but many will not, with the financial demands of securing services for those prone to ADHD growing ever greater and the struggle to find time ever harder.

More often than not the little time we have at home is not taken up with play or quality time with our kids, but with other forms of work – chores, housework, gardening, financial planning – the other 'out-of-work' responsibilities necessary to support a family. In this context it is not only practical but rational to keep our kids busy by giving them access to hours of television, video and computer games, all of which are safer and more convenient activities than going out. But letting children spend all that time in front of a screen does more than encourage obesity – it also means less time to develop the imagination that comes from creative play as well as the play that burns off excess energy. Neither does spending time with a screen help to build the relationships and social skills that come from playing with other children or adults and learning to get on with them. For some children, lack of interactive play with others can also stunt their language development – and this may have particular implications for boys.

Compared to girls, boys take longer to acquire language and interpersonal skills, so it's even more important for them to have the chance to develop and improve them. There may be fewer opportunities to play with other children, while the prevalence of smaller families means they have a narrower range of people to which to relate. Added to this is the decline in the kind of blue-collar work culture that used to provide opportunities for teenage boys to develop interpersonal skills in a traditionally masculine way – maybe as a labourer working in a team, or a delegate lobbying in a trade union, or a player competing with other adult males through sport.

Boys and schooling

It's also become harder for 'boys to be boys' in schools. Legitimate concerns about harassment and public liability mean there's less scope for things like camps and outdoor education. I am aware of some public schools where teachers have stopped taking their class outside the school gates because of the mountain of paperwork that needs to be completed. In our attempt to safeguard against risk, we may also be removing opportunities for boys to mature through calculated risk-taking. Further, the schoolyard behaviours that were acceptable for a boy a generation ago (like boisterous play or pranks) are clamped down on in many schools because of potential risk.

Meanwhile, increased class sizes, more students with needs and heavier teaching workloads make it harder for teachers to include the kind of active learning projects that allow children to move around in the classroom and practice relationship-building with others. As any teacher will tell you, the larger the class of students in a classroom, the more the traditional 'rows of desks' learning style is the only one possible. This may suit some subjects and some students, but the post-Internet generation makes greater demands for stimulation in learning than perhaps any previous generation. Added to this, the competition for future employment, the drive for standardised education and the desire to gain top marks in Year 12 places pressure on teachers to put 'content' before the individual student's needs and use a 'cookie cutter' approach to teaching. If we try to make all children meet standard educational expectations, we ignore individual differences in the way children behave and learn.

Increasing problems with discipline and low attendance also have an effect. In schools where high numbers of children take days off, teachers have to work overtime to help these students catch up on the days when they turn up. If discipline is an issue, teachers have to spend more of their class time trying to maintain order. And if you teach in the secondary environment, where contact time with each class is low, then the ability to build positive relationships is limited. Together this will eat into the possibility for more creative and engaging activities in the classroom. Where this challenge is felt most acutely is in secondary schools where the whole school is run on a senior school timeline, which usually results in lots of lesson changes and a different teacher for every subject. This can be very traumatic for students adjusting from primary school, and can present an emotional and organisational challenge to those in their early teens when stability in routines and relationships are so important. Again, young people who struggle with ADHD will feel these challenges more acutely.

Taken together, all these pressures make it harder for schools to help boys be boys. Given that so many jobs are now sedentary or involve little physical activity, and that education encourages more disciplined and focused study, these constraints on boys may only get worse. I say this because since the 1980s Australia's education policy has been to link educational goals to vocational skills. This, along with the growth in information technology (IT), means education increasingly encourages IT, tertiary-trained industry and white-collar skills that are more passive. Jobs in these areas can mean a lot of sitting still and concentrating at a computer, working with your head (not your hands) and drawing on good interpersonal and communication skills. As blue-collar work has dwindled, there is less space for people who abound in physical energy, are intuitive rather than logical, and work through challenges by doing rather than reflecting. So the new benchmark for behaviour in our classrooms is increasingly based on the traditional model of the hard-working, studious female student, and because schools are primarily geared towards a one-size-fits-all standard of success, success means students need to be passive and compliant.

Once upon a time, kids who found it hard to conform in the classroom could sometimes stick it out because there were more ways to compensate by letting off steam outside school. Then, if you couldn't put up with school any longer, you left

In the long term it is probably more useful to think about how to make society more accepting of difference than how to diagnose more

and found a job. But with fewer blue-collar jobs available, stubbornly high youth unemployment and a pressure to keep kids at school longer, there aren't many career opportunities for boys who are active, inattentive and impulsive and don't fancy a working life pinned to a chair or standing behind a counter. Some may do well in sport, running their own business or in the armed forces, but many become unemployed or stuck in the lowest-paid unskilled jobs. Research shows that if we keep boys at school longer, the quality and quantity of work they later have improves. However, we must also ask what it is about schools that make more boys so desperate to leave – so that we can give them more reason to stay.

These trends don't make it easy for many boys generally, and may be behind many of the problems they now face. Of course, for children with hyperactive and impulsive behaviours, these pressures are felt more acutely. As my experience with boys' respite camps made so clear, boys with ADHD are now part of the growing number of children being labelled 'problem kids' who, a generation or two ago, would have just been seen as 'different' or going through an active stage of a boy's normal development. We have changed as a society, and these changes have made hyperactive and impulsive behaviour more conspicuous.

The ADHD gender gap

Given the nature of the link between ADHD and drug treatment (which I explained in a previous chapter), it will come as no surprise to discover that drug use for ADHD is usually much higher for boys than it is for girls. While figures once suggested that about five boys for every one girl were diagnosed and treated with drugs for ADHD, this ratio has since dropped closer to three to one. This is not due to boys being given fewer drugs, rather it is because more girls are being diagnosed and treated as ADHD becomes better known.

Yet an ADHD gender gap still remains, and some experts suggest that it could be partly explained by the way ADHD is studied and diagnosed. Fewer studies are done using girls, for instance, and because the criteria for diagnosing ADHD in the US and Australia were developed using boys, this could create a male bias, resulting in more boys being diagnosed. Does this then mean boys and girls need different criteria for an ADHD diagnosis? Maybe, but in the long term it is probably more useful to think about how to make society more accepting of difference than how to diagnose more.

The most common difference between boys and girls with ADHD is that boys tend to show more hyperactive behaviour, while girls are more likely to have problems with inattention. As Dr Lawrence Diller puts it, 'boys tend to act out, while girls tend to act in'. Due to this, it may be that many girls with the disorder go undiagnosed, and struggle at school – especially high school. Interestingly, when girls with ADHD are hyperactive, they have even greater problems being accepted than boys do, and are less likely to have friends – which reinforces the strength of the different social expectations on boys and girls that start at birth. The different ways that we bring up boys and girls go beyond dressing one in pink and the other in blue. We encourage one to explore the space around them, while the other we dress in a skirt, and tell to stay home. As teenagers, one group is urged to be assertive and active, while the other is told to be supportive of others.

> *'If a society puts half its children in dresses and skirts but warns them not to move in ways that reveal their underpants, while putting the other half in jeans and overalls and encouraging them to climb trees and play ball and other outdoor games; if later during adolescence the half that has worn trousers is exhorted to "eat like a growing boy" while the half in skirts is warned to watch its weight and not get fat ... then these two groups of people will grow to be biologically as well as socially different. Their muscles will be different, as will their reflexes, posture, arms, legs, and feet, hand–eye coordination, spatial perception and so on.'*
>
> **Dr G. Vines, physical education and dance expert**

Clearly, if we treat each group differently, then we must expect that eventually they'll be physically as well as socially different. This raises the possibility that the way we raise children can shape the way their bodies and brains develop. This alone questions the prominent idea that children with ADHD are born with a physical difference that causes social problems. In short, could it be the other way around? Could nurturing play a part in the development of a physical difference? If that is the case, are there mixed messages that we are sending from birth for boys to be active in order to be masculine, but passive in order to succeed at school and work? Is this setting the scene for ADHD?

Just how much gender has an influence on the way parents treat their children is still open to debate, and more research is needed. From my own experience and from looking at recent social trends, I get the feeling that expectations about gender and social roles do influence families. A common view is shown in the comments by two of the boys in my study, Leon and Stephen, who both claimed their sister also had ADHD, but it was different to theirs. Let's start with Leon, who opened this chapter.

> He was a stocky, blond, 14-year-old who talked with a fast slur. It always amazed me how a boy who seemed so congenial got into so much trouble – perhaps it was out of frustration with the difficulty he had in putting his thoughts into words. On a couple of occasions, Leon spoke of how his behaviour had deteriorated since his parents had separated. You got the feeling that the presence of his father had helped keep him in line, but when the discipline was left to his mother, Leon had trouble taking her seriously. 'It's just like if Dad was home I would do everything right, like if I got into trouble Dad would give me a backhander or something like that... so now it's like Mum can't do anything, I just laugh at her.'
>
> But he went on to confide that his mum 'almost had a nervous breakdown and that kind of stuff. …' (see Leon's full comment on page 102).

Leon was at a loss as to how he could fix this situation – and his story highlights the distress that many children with ADHD feel when they have the insight to know they're doing something wrong but feel helpless to change it. This can be a real source of misery and frustration.

Meanwhile, 14-year-old Stephen felt that because he had only a mild case of ADHD he wasn't a typical example. He was adamant, however, that his whole family had the disorder:

'My sister has a tiny case, she's not as bad as me, and it doesn't show up on the tests. My mum has it but she's never been tested because her parents didn't believe in it, and Dad's pretty cool, he probably has it, but no-one knows. You inherit ADHD from your family, you see ...'

Comments like these show that not only do some families use ADHD to label both their sons and their daughters (regardless of whether they show extreme hyperactive or inattentive behaviours or not), but that they also accept that boys have more problem behaviour.

Boys and literacy

Something that might offer insight into ADHD and gender is recent research into the problems boys face with literacy at school. In general, studies show that boys don't perform as well as girls, and find English less interesting. Some approaches have tried to include more active or aggressive texts, but this has had minimal success (and often excludes girls). Instead, more recent approaches to teaching literacy have tried to counteract the idea that being good at English is a 'girl thing' because it involves reflection, talking about feelings, and sitting around reading rather than being active. To make English more appealing to boys, schools have tried putting more emphasis on activity in class, excursions, and incorporating popular culture, computers and electronic media. At least from the indications so far, this seems to be having some success.

Why this is relevant to ADHD is that it shows the power that gender can have on a young person's learning. If some boys fail in certain subjects because they clash with ideas of masculinity, it is not enough to blame a father who never touches a book; we also need to find ways to make boys feel male *and* literate. If this applies to learning, why then might the same thing not apply to behaviour in the classroom? Boys prone to overactivity may also feel that being active is part of being male, and will find it harder to tone down their behaviour. If we just accept the cycle that Dad was a 'ratbag' and the son is just following in his footsteps, we will make little progress. Neither will we move forward if we try to take away the space for boys to be boys. But if we can come up with ways to make them feel active and male while they learn and live, we might start getting somewhere.

Why boys?

Whether it be caused by nature, nurture, or both, it may be that the biology of boys is different and that the body chemistry of some makes them more overactive. As a result, these boys find it hard to rein in behaviours that once might have been an asset for survival. As ADHD diagnosis and treatment has become better known and the expectations of our schools have changed, it seems that boys with active and resistant behaviour have drawn attention to themselves. This at least in part explains why there are more boys diagnosed with ADHD.

As for girls, it may be that both sexes have similar biological propensities and that ADHD is just as likely in both – but because the checklist for diagnosing the disorder came from studies of six-year-old boys, it may not be as effective for assessing girls (and that's why they're diagnosed less often). It might also be that both boys and girls are biologically similar in respect to ADHD, but their different upbringing helps explain why girls tend to be diagnosed at an older age. We bring up girls to be less active, more emotive and better at social communication. As a result, they're less likely to be identified by a diagnostic checklist that stresses overactivity, impulsivity and problems in social settings. Instead, those who are diagnosed tend to be diagnosed at a later age, when problems of inattention emerge because of the higher academic demands of high school.

It is important to realise that so far we don't have enough research to prove any of these explanations. My own view is that a complex web of social changes in our work, school, family, gender roles and even in patterns of recreation has had a real impact on boys in recent years. This impact has been especially hard on boys with an ADHD predisposition, and in many ways this makes ADHD a window into recent changes and priorities in Australian society – a matter that will be further discussed in a later chapter.

Key points

- Different social expectations on boys may contribute to the greater diagnosis of ADHD among boys.
- Boys are more likely to be diagnosed with ADHD in primary school for hyperactivity, while girls are more likely to be diagnosed for inattention in early secondary school.
- Boys are struggling more with recent changes in expectations in behaviours, school, recreation and work.
- Boys prone to ADHD will find these recent changes harder to adapt to than most.

6

ADHD in schools

'I guess there isn't really a way to make school better for kids [with ADHD], otherwise they would have thought it up and used it by now. It's just been the same system of schooling since there has been school, sit down and write, add and subtract … you'd have to change the system,' said Billy (who is 13).

'And they can't change the system?' I asked.

'Nah, it costs too much and they wouldn't want to anyway.'

'Why not?'

'Cause it's up to the individual to change … you can't change school to make it fit everybody.'

A major idea behind this book is that past responses to ADHD have been too medical and too incomplete. Mostly, effort has gone into getting a child to fit their surroundings through medical or other means. The problem is that it is not only the fault of the child that they have a troubled life at school. Environment can make a big difference for young people with ADHD. Yet rather than ask what schools might be doing wrong, we say the problem is mostly with the child, and label him or her as the troublemaker. One of the major purposes of this book is to crack this notion open and look at both sides of the ADHD coin – the individual and the social. And since the main social bottleneck through which young people pass is the school, the classroom cannot be left out of a fuller consideration of ADHD.

While there are plenty of big issues to consider about ADHD and school, we cannot ignore the fact that teachers and parents are desperate for help in the here and now. If teachers are to help students with ADHD they need behavioural strategies to create the time, and learning strategies to make the space for big-picture progress. If all of one's energy and time is lost on behaviour management, there is little left for finding ways of teaching and learning that suit individual student needs. While some educators claim that relevant and rigorous learning captures a student's attention so that behavioural problems disappear, in my experience I've found that things work best with practical strategies to support both behaviour and learning. For this reason, I provide 100 helpful hints for teaching students with ADHD.

100 helpful hints for teachers

Seating

1   Sit students away from distractions.
2   Have a seating plan.
3   Set up desks with space around each and try to avoid seating plans where the student is looking directly at others.
4   Sit the student next to a good role model/buddy and reward both together for on-task behaviour and work.

5   Allow students to straddle or sit backwards on their chair while still facing the teacher.

6   Provide the student with space where they can work but still move (e.g. work at a desk standing up).

7   Allow for a two-site plan (one area away from distraction and another where the student can let off steam without distracting others).

8   Occasionally give students the opportunity to rest or 'veg' on the condition that they do not disturb others.

Behaviour

9   Make every lesson a fresh start for you *and* the students.

10   Have a staged behaviour management plan for your classes, print it off and get students to stick it inside the front cover of their books (and refer to it regularly).

11   Be quick to use this plan to identify when 'good' students breach it; you need to not only be even-handed, but be seen to be even-handed.

12   Explain the rationale of your decisions to the whole class as fair: 'I did this for X last week, I am doing the same with you today.'

13   Develop secret code words with the ADHD student to signal that behaviour is escalating into an unhelpful cycle, without the rest of the class knowing.

14   Regularly use hand or sound signals with the whole class to reinforce requests for desired behaviour.

15   Use the same key phrases to show the urgency of your requests (e.g. 'Quiet thanks', becomes 'You should be quiet now so I can speak', becomes 'I am talking, you must stop').

16   Avoid putting the student's name on the board for bad behaviour.

17 Break down the school's behaviour management plan into small steps, so students can track how close they are to being in trouble (e.g. an in-class card system or points system).

18 Watch the particular difficulties your student with ADHD experiences and how they vary in time and place. Try to minimise things that act as triggers or that increase the gap between what the student can do and what the environment demands of them.

19 Watch your students' eyes and facial expressions closely – they can often be indicators for when they are getting 'wound up'. Try to have an errand or two up your sleeve to get them out of the classroom for a purposeful break.

20 Plan for likely behaviour problems, so you have a couple of choices with logical consequences ready, and present the student with a choice.

21 Move away from the student and give them a set time to think about their choice (i.e. do not escalate the situation by standing over them until they choose).

22 Make sure they never avoid the logical consequences they choose.

23 Never accept ADHD as an excuse. If students are honest they will admit that they always choose, it's just that the medication makes it easier. Try to help them create a situation where it is easier to choose appropriately.

24 If possible, take a walk with the student to discuss problems of conflict and anger; never face them toe-to-toe.

25 When talking with the student in tense situations, try to avoid escalating the problem by giving both parties a way to save face (even if you have to apologise first when you were not in the wrong).

26 Set up a system where a student can self-monitor on-task behaviour and can check this off with you/their buddy to earn rewards.

27 Set up a system where students can self-select time-out to calm down (e.g. they hand you a card which allows them to go outside for five minutes).

28 Make a behaviour contract that is very specific about exactly which actions cause problems and map out rewards/ consequences.

29 When you make a contract, make sure the goals are achievable and the reward is given ASAP, then extend the goal after each success.

30 Ensure rewards are immediate.

31 Consciously plan more relaxed times in lessons.

32 If a student has had a really bad day, let them work off some of the logical consequences of their actions by making positive contributions to the class (e.g. cleaning up, making something for the class, a formal apology, etc).

Lesson planning

33 Use a similar pattern to start each lesson and help students settle into the lesson.

34 Allow time for students to wind down after breaks or group work sessions (i.e. don't move straight from play to silent reading).

35 Try to do similar types of work at similar times each week.

36 Have a set schedule for submitting work each week.

37 Try to do activities that require more attention in the morning.

38 Switch between mental and physical activities.

39 Allow oral assessment.

40 Allow plenty of opportunities to practise with peers before assessment.

41 Use peer tutoring.

42 Have a teacher buddy nearby who is informed of what you are doing in class and to whom you can send the student to work, if all else fails in your class.

43 Teach around themes and make the links between different aspects very explicit.
44 Minimise teacher talk time.

Lesson delivery

45 Pause regularly when you speak to keep students interested.
46 Tell stories or create a sense of mystery.
47 Use all five senses to teach whenever possible.
48 Stand near students with ADHD when instructing them.
49 Get a student's attention back through an unrelated question that interests them before asking a question about their work.
50 When using PowerPoint or OHPs, use colour extensively and hide information that is not being directly used at the time.
51 Make the transitions between parts of the lesson explicit.
52 Repeat lesson objectives several times.
53 Use instructions that contain one concept at a time.
54 If a student asks for assistance (and you are with another student) give the student a set time by which you will get to them (and make sure you do so).
55 If possible, get all students to come and seek assistance at the front of the class so you can both help them and monitor their progress.
56 Vary the way you ask for responses in class (as well as who gets to answer).
57 Get students into the habit of all thinking for a few seconds before they answer.

Student work

58 Have a book in which a student can draw or doodle while listening in class.
59 Encourage students to think out loud.
60 Provide examples of successful student work with scaffolding of what was good about it and the structure/process it uses.

61   Colour-code actions consistently across handouts (e.g. red 'think box', green 'write box', etc.) and underline, colour or label the important parts of assignments.

62   Break down questions/tasks into steps (don't assume that what has to be done is self-evident).

63   Try to avoid remedial approaches and plan intellectually demanding tasks.

64   Teach different methods of solving problems based on different ways of thinking, and allow students to experiment with their preferred model.

65   During reading or whole-class work, move around the class and subtly point to the place on the page that the class is up to.

66   Where possible, provide texts on audiotape.

67   Teach students to use colour coding to organise their ideas and to put their ideas together (e.g. for concept charts or essay writing).

68   Get students to paraphrase instructions in their own words.

69   Modify assessments to enable student success, or reduce the number of assessment pieces required.

70   Look for ways to assess creatively or by one criteria/outcome and do not assess everything at once.

Organisation skills

71   Set aside space on the board to record homework, class rules and calendar items; do not move it and refer to it explicitly in class.

72   Provide students with a 'to do' list in a plastic folder on their desk and update it regularly.

73   Consider providing students with a keyring USB that is attached to something they will never lose (and save all their work to this).

74   Set aside a special place for books, materials, etc., and monitor this area.

75 Give the students classtime to organise their materials.

76 Use colour coding for subjects and give out new materials pre-punched for folders.

77 Give students pre-printed copies of notes from the board.

78 Explicitly teach skills like note-taking, summarising and organising ideas.

79 Provide partially complete lesson overviews and conclude the lesson with the students filling in the gaps.

80 If students have real difficulty, set up an organisation plan for each teacher to sign (with diary use, materials brought, homework finished, work in class) and use this in two-week bursts with a reward (have a break between bursts and don't use this for behaviour management purposes).

Resources

81 Use technology where possible (e.g. computers, calculators, CD-ROMs, palm-organisers).

82 Vary the mediums used in a lesson (e.g. DVD, pictures, music, computers).

83 Purchase textbooks that are colourful, have clear layout and are not text-heavy (also be conscious of the complexity of words used).

84 Try to use textbooks that have a clear flow of ideas, use the actual textbooks (not photocopies of sections) and try not to jump around in the book.

85 If you have the option of a CD-ROM or DVD for a text, use it by getting the student with ADHD and a buddy to work online.

86 If you can book a computer room and have the whole class using DVD resources on a network, do it as regularly as you can.

Communication with home

87   Let students listen to their own music with headphones during class work times.

88   Maintain frequent contact with home to provide positive feedback and check that school messages are getting through.

89   Check that work is being put in the student's diary.

90   Produce a term overview of when assignments are due and make sure it gets home to parents.

Social skills/Self-esteem needs

91   Always be looking for opportunities to give positive feedback and to praise strengths.

92   Never use the ADHD label as a negative term in front of other students (even if the student with ADHD does).

93   Avoid 'put-down' humour or sarcasm: at best, students with poor social skills will act as though they understand (but just get hurt); at worst, they will imitate it because everyone laughed (and get in even more trouble).

94   Model good conflict resolution and democratic decision-making in class and through group activities.

95   Use class votes or the votes of the people sitting around the student with difficulty to decide if the student should be moved (use this as a very early warning, not in place of logical consequence choices).

96   Give students specific responsibilities for the class and publicly encourage them for completing these responsibilities. Set the student up with an older student tutor to help them in your subject area.

97   Plan for group work regularly but change groups around so that the student with ADHD is not always with the same classmates.

98　Be wary of group activities that the ADHD student cannot do as the group may turn on them and blame them for failure (this will quickly blow up into a problem).

99　If you send out a student with ADHD for extra special education support, try to arrange to send along strong students as well for additional (higher-level) support so the ADHD student avoids the stigma of always being sent out.

100　Work hard to find out about the student's interests outside of school, and keep up discussions about their successes in this area.

Many of these strategies will not be new to teachers, yet as experienced teachers will recognise, it is very difficult to get them all right at the same time. The pressure on teacher work, class sizes and behaviour management issues see teachers fall away from using these strategies at times. It is easy to say that if we can engage students, behaviour management will not be a problem; it is much harder to make this a reality. A renewed effort to use these strategies (which will benefit all students) can make a difference for the students with ADHD in your classroom.

ADHD and school – the big picture

Children and adolescents with ADHD have a high risk of underachieving at school. According to Western Australian research, 35–50 percent of children with ADHD have to repeat a year (compared to 10 percent of children without ADHD). These students are also more likely to be suspended or expelled. Is it possible that ADHD has become a way to explain the growing numbers of children who no longer fit in Australia's classrooms? In the rest of this chapter, I will consider a number of changing influences on schooling that make it harder for students with ADHD.

Education and the economy

The first such influence is what Australian education expert, Professor John Smyth, calls the 'welding of education onto the economy.' What this phrase refers to is that Australian education hasn't escaped the effects of recent economic changes. Now that we're part of a global economy, we need a skilled workforce to help us remain economically competitive. Our schools are the key to preparing young people for work and protecting our economy in the future. As a result, education policy now has a stronger focus on using limited resources to produce a steady supply of suitably qualified workers. This is a reflection of current political thinking: the neo-liberal push to improve efficiency and productivity in all areas of policy.

These changes in Australian education have had a real impact on schools, affecting both the curriculum and the level of support for teachers and students. As governments have become less involved in providing services to schools, there has been a reduction in support officers in public schools. This has added to the administrative load on teachers, who now have less time and energy to meet the needs of specific students – including those with ADHD. The frustration parents have with this lack of support can cause tension and conflict between families and schools, which does nothing to promote successful learning.

One part of this shift has been for both primary and secondary schools students to have more standardised testing and assessment geared to a narrower range of vocational goals. This way, governments can be sure that schools are supplying the market with the skilled workers it needs, and it helps young people get jobs.

The problem is that by putting increasing pressure on schools to teach each student according to one standard, there's less flexibility for teaching children according to their personality, social background or individual needs. Not all students are suited to a one-size-fits-all curriculum, and this can be a real problem. Depending on their background, home life or experience, some children will do well – but some will not. A child with tertiary-educated parents (who may work in the new information economy) will fit more easily into a school system geared toward these values. Meanwhile, a child whose parents work in a declining manufacturing industry will find it harder to learn what they need to do to succeed. This means that unless there's some positive discrimination to make the classroom a more level playing field, many children will struggle to succeed.

By positive discrimination, I mean teaching students overtly about what it takes to do well in schools. University of Nottingham Professor (and ex-South Australian school principal) Pat Thomson talks about the 'virtual schoolbag' that every child brings with them. Some children arrive on the first day with a virtual schoolbag of acquired skills that sets them up for success at school – others do not. For many students with ADHD, they arrive with very empty virtual schoolbags despite their parents' best efforts. The onus is on our schools to teach these skills to these students so that they have the same toolkit as their peers, as well as to make time to link what they have brought from home in their virtual schoolbags to the curriculum in meaningful ways. This both values the student and equips him or her for success in the future. Such an approach does not sit well with a standards approach to education that assumes a level playing field and identifies any gaps in skills or knowledge as the fault of the student.

Education policy now has a stronger focus on using limited resources to produce a steady supply of suitably qualified workers

The other problem posed by the standards approach in the classroom is that most people still believe education is about preparing people as citizens. While getting a post-school job or going on to further education is important, education is about teaching young people how to earn a living and how to live a life. This is a problem for a standardised curriculum because people's lives are not standardised, and standardisation makes it hard to value qualities such as individuality, creativity and community spirit. The risk of a narrower and standardised curriculum is that it restricts education – it puts limits on who gets educated, how and about what.

The education squeeze

As these new priorities put the squeeze on education, some students get squeezed out. This raises an important question: who's responsible for those who don't meet these new criteria? It is here that the growth in ADHD provides a fascinating insight. The ADHD label and drug treatment can account for the students whose hyperactivity doesn't fit these new standards, as well as explain those whose inattention means they don't do well in standardised tests. In other words, *the label can be a convenient way of explaining the growing number of young people who don't fit new behavioural, educational and social standards.* No wonder the medical theory of ADHD can be so appealing.

Rather than look at how issues like high youth unemployment, large class sizes, changing school curricula, and less funding for schools might affect some young people, ADHD focuses on the faults of the young person. It's also a useful way of depoliticising the effects of recent funding cuts on education – that is, by putting all the focus on the problems within the individual, we risk being distracted from the challenges that they share and, more importantly, what might be causing them.

In my work with young people with ADHD, a common theme is that they do not feel they fit in at school – and that they are part of a school system that makes things harder. The story of 13-year-old Darren is typical of how children with ADHD struggle at school.

'When I started off primary school I was hyperactive. I couldn't sit still and … like … at school I just didn't want to be there very much. But I started school off well, like I had a good teacher, but then in Year Two I had a teacher who didn't like me, so I took a real dislike to her and so that didn't work well at all, and they took me out of that primary school and put me in another primary school. I'm told I did alright in Year Three but I can't remember it that much, but my mum says I stuffed up big time at the end of the year …

'It was a sports day or somethin', and me and some friends were writing stuff on the walls and that … and we got into a lot of shit … and yeah … from there on, first thing at the start of the year, I find out straight away that me and four other students are being made to sit down the front so the teacher can keep a watch on us … and we had to earn these little blocks for being good so that we could go out at recess and lunch. I just thought, "This is bullshit". Every time a teacher gave me a hassle like I'd give her one back twice as bad … and that didn't work out for me at all 'cause pretty much the same thing happened the next year … and I resented that and refused to cooperate.

'So in Year Six … I had a teacher, she was expecting trouble from me from the start and she went out of her way to make sure to sorta say, "I'm not going to put up with any of your crap, you'll come into line and do what I say." I started off in first term really well and she came up to me and said, "Why you being so good?", and I said "I don't wanna get in trouble"… and she said, "Well I was expecting you to not be behaving so well considering all your previous years at this school."

'But I mean that year we had like one teacher Monday, Tuesday, Thursday, Friday, and another on Wednesday. And I don't know what happened there but me and this teacher on Wednesday just didn't kick off. Like the punishment system came along somewhere along the line, and you had to go and sit at a desk away from the rest of the class and fill out a contract before you rejoined the class ... and just about every second Wednesday I was in there filling out a contract.'

Darren said that he had settled better at his high school, Westside High, but felt bitter towards his previous schools and teachers.

Teachers I spoke with also had clear opinions about the place of ADHD in school and the problems it presented. At Eastside High, Margaret, a teacher who was respected by all the boys in the study, offered this insight into children with ADHD in schools:

'If the student doesn't have a trusting relationship with their teacher, they will act out. All kids will act out if they have something on their mind. Definitely, the kids with ADHD have to have someone they can talk to ... and preferably to every teacher they come in contact with. I think it has been really fortunate that if there is anything happening, the kids have the same three teachers for at least two lessons a day ... and we can build up the relationships to help support them because they have a whole lot of fears about what's going on. I think it has been disappointing that some people have not given any credence to ADHD, have not even given the kids positive feedback for the small improvements they have made ... and I think the kids themselves resent that. One boy in particular has nearly been in tears because he has been kicked out from a particular lesson, and he said, "Fuckin' hell – can't they see I am trying my fuckin' hardest? What do they want from me?"'

Margaret went on: 'My initial impression, like a lot of teachers, was of ADHD as a very fashionable cover for students who have had either poor parenting or umm ... some trauma in their life, that they were acting out and either had no self-discipline or would not accept external discipline.'

'What gave you this initial impression of ADHD?' I asked.

'Well, I saw some horrific behaviour on television programs and read some books on ADHD, and I guess there was a query in my mind. But I suppose that I was convinced when I saw how dramatically the drugs change their behaviour. But I'd be worried if ADHD was overly diagnosed, because there are still students that just need really clear boundaries and won't settle down.'

I asked, 'Have there been things in the school that make it harder to help kids with ADHD?'

'I think the decline in the status of teachers has a significant impact. You have to work so hard all the time to earn the students' respect, and for kids with ADHD it makes it even harder for them to know where the line is.

'I think it is also a decline in parenting, and people wanting someone else to own the problem and own the solution ... and we have a whole generation of parents who do not commit themselves to being involved in their child's education. It's the spending time at home and actually supervising homework ... it is switching off televisions ... it's having meals together ...'

Margaret laughed as she said, 'I'm not usually this conservative ... yeah, but it's those kinds of structures that support behaviour.'

As part of my research, I also spoke to the special education staff in the schools. When I spoke to Tammy, the special education coordinator at a high school in Adelaide's Western Suburbs (a low-income area), she made it very clear what exacerbated the problems with ADHD:

'There is just not enough time and resources,' she said, explaining that she had only five free periods each week to assess and develop individualised plans for 40 students with specific educational needs.

'That's amazing,' I replied.

'That's why I'm not doing it next year.'

'What could help special educators meet the needs of students with ADHD?' I asked.

'Reduce class sizes; provide more teacher training – not just information about the condition, but also strategies to cope with it; and, I think, getting them out of the classroom.'

Tammy continued, '… if you have an ADD kid and you can get them out occasionally and into things, give them a breather from the classroom, but at the same time still be challenged, that's sometimes all it needs. But all that is time and money, it always comes down to that.'

This point is picked up by education specialist Professor Roger Slee (former Deputy Director General of the Queensland Department of Education and now Dean of Education at McGill University in Montreal). He argues that as government policies call for higher retention rates in schools, and as the pressures on teachers grow, discipline policies will increasingly be used to hide the inability of schools to meet rapidly changing educational expectations. In other words, a focus on managing behaviour in schools will draw attention away from the behaviour of school management. As discipline policies in schools shift from punishment to treatment, there's more potential to identify individual students as the problem, rather than the school, and I would suggest that ADHD neatly fits within this shift.

'As the contexts of young people and the expectations for their schooling become more complex, the greater is their [i.e. Australian state education departments'] determination to establish explanations which locate the problem within individual, aberrant students and the solution in therapeutic interventions of expert professionals.'

Professor Roger Slee

When one considers American research that shows that parents only seek out an ADHD diagnosis after giving up on getting support from schools, there is reason to believe that there are not only more young people not fitting in at school, but also that more are being told that they are the problem. With narrowing expectations on children in the classroom, the pressures of less time and resources on teachers, as well as Australia increasingly welding education onto the economy, it's becoming ever easier to think about differences in children as deficiencies, disorders – or even economic dangers.

In a tougher educational climate, ADHD can be a humane way of handling the students not brilliant enough to meet the tighter standards for educational success, **Not only are more young people not fitting in at school, more are being told that they are the problem** but not damaged enough to meet criteria for disability assistance. As Australian schools are pushed further away from the principles of equality, public interest and social justice, and towards individualism, the economy and standardisation, the medical theory of ADHD has the popular credibility to explain why there are a growing number of students who do not fit the system. Not only that, ADHD also provides drug treatment, a tool that can pacify them to fit the very standards and structures that would alienate them.

Could it be that Australia is now more interested in individual conformity than it is in why people some are missing out in the first place? Perhaps it is timely to reflect again on the sentiment commonly attributed to Samuel Johnson:

'One should measure the civilisation of a nation not by the achievements of its greatest, but by how it treats its most vulnerable.'

Key points

- Young people spend the vast majority of their waking life at school, so teachers and schools are in the frontline with ADHD.
- Drugs do not make kids learn better; it lets them choose. It is important to supplement pills with educational strategies.
- Recent changes in schooling to teach to the standard, rather than to the individual, result in more kids that do not fit, and young people with ADHD are among the most affected by these changes.
- ADHD provides an endorsed rationale and humane response to the growing number of students squeezed out of schooling.
- Kids do not fail school because they do not understand schoolwork; they fail because schools do not understand how they work.

7

ADHD and society

'In the reality of the workaday world, the individual is expected to cope with society to a greater degree than society is expected to cope with the individual. Children with negative behaviours get classified and treated; adults get fired or arrested.'

Professor R. Smelter, US educational expert

If you are reading this chapter and your child is diagnosed ADHD, then odds are that you are probably Anglo-Saxon, don't watch SBS, earn less than $35,000 a year and your child is a boy. Why is that?

In this chapter I will explore how ADHD is viewed differently by ethnicity, income and cultural background. I will also look at the differences in ADHD internationally and ponder why drug use for ADHD has been prominent in Australia, New Zealand and North America, but less so in other Western nations.

Despite all the fuss about ADHD, little attention has been given to why ADHD has exploded in some parts of some societies but not in others. If you accept the idea that ADHD is a physical difference within the human gene pool, you would think that ADHD would be found relatively evenly across all peoples. Admittedly, some families would have a stronger genetic leaning toward ADHD, but you would not expect huge variations according to ethnicity, class or gender. However, this has been the case, and it is another reason why medical questions about ADHD are not alone enough to understand ADHD. Instead, we need to look at the social factors that may be at work, and try to understand why there's so much variation in diagnosis according to where children live, their ethnic background, how affluent their families are, and whether they are boys or girls – variations which, so far, medical research can't explain.

Does ethnic background make a difference?

In Australia, children from Asian or indigenous backgrounds seem less likely to be diagnosed with ADHD. Not enough research has been completed to make the variations between different ethnic groups clear, but it may be that different attitudes in different cultures have an impact. It's hard to generalise, but compared to Anglo-Saxon families in Australia, for instance, attitudes to discipline in many Asian families can be different – there may be higher expectations of children's behaviour and more emphasis on being reserved and controlled. There may also be a tradition of relying on the family for support rather than turning to health professionals for help with family problems.

Another possibility is that when a child's ethnic background is already associated – rightly or wrongly – with overactive or difficult behaviour, then simply belonging to that ethnic group may be considered enough of an explanation without having to go looking for a label or diagnosis. In the minds of some people, stereotypes about being indigenous, for instance, might be enough reason to explain a child's hyperactivity or difficulty with concentration.

However, there are grounds to believe that the situation is different among Maori children in New Zealand. Although there is a lack of data on prevalence among Maori children, it is estimated that there is little variance in prevalence with the rest of the population. Again, the explanation for similarities or differences between different ethnic groups isn't clear, but possibly a relatively more successful reconciliation between Maori and Western cultures has enabled a greater adoption of an ADHD model originating from the United States.

In the US, ADHD is primarily a white, upper middle-class phenomenon, with African-American children and minority groups less likely to be labelled with ADHD and given prescription drugs. Given that in the US ethnic background is often linked to poverty, it's hard to know whether cultural factors are making a difference or whether it's the lack of money for health care. With African-American families there may also be a reluctance to resort to drugs, given the impact of drug abuse in their communities. Yet there's also evidence that while African-American children are less likely to get a diagnosis and treatment, they're more likely than Caucasian children to be identified with ADHD-like behaviours. This coincides with some evidence that minority-group children in the US have to show higher levels of symptoms before they get referred for help. Put simply, cultural differences can make what is unacceptable to one group appear acceptable to another.

Different cultures also have different views on medicine and science. It may be that the idea of ADHD as a medical problem is not readily accepted by some cultures either inside or outside Australia because they don't have such blind faith in scientific research. Alternatively, it may be that in some cultures and societies an unquestioning trust in science and a tendency to look for quick fixes may make it hard to see ADHD as anything other than a medical problem fixable with drugs.

When it comes to understanding more about ADHD and ethnic cultures in Australia, it would be nice to think that our cultural diversity has helped us accept a range of views on ADHD. Yet research in this area is almost non-existent. Perhaps to understand ADHD and ethnicity, we need to think about it through the example of shifts in Australian cultural attitudes since the 1950s. Until then, a strict White Australia Policy limited the immigration of anyone who wasn't white, Protestant and British. Even when the need to boost the workforce after World War Two opened the doors to European immigrants and transformed Australia's cultural mix, the national identity and values remained very British. But from the 1970s onwards, this changed dramatically under Labor and Liberal governments, when waves of immigrants arrived from Asia and the Middle East. This trend reached a peak in 1993, when Australia proclaimed itself a multicultural country.

However, the position of recent conservative governments has reflected a clear swing back to more traditional values and identity in Australia. What this may mean is that it makes Australia's mainstream culture more open to trends in other conservative Anglo cultures, such as the US. It could be that as Australia mirrored a shift towards conservatism in American politics, it also embraced the pragmatic, quick-fix, medical view of ADHD (so prominent in the US). While non-Anglo ethnic groups in Australia may look at ADHD through a different cultural lens, the growth in ADHD could be because Anglo-Australians are more open to accepting an American cultural viewpoint.

Whatever the reason, it is clear that in most cases ADHD diagnosis and drug use varies greatly by ethnicity. But there remain some unanswered questions. Is this due to different cultural responses to behaviour, science or drug use? Is it that the biological problem underpinning ADHD is common to everyone, and that ethnic communities need better ADHD education and services? Or is it that you have to be a white Anglo-Saxon male to be diagnosed ADHD? Regardless, we need to find out more and we need to reflect on the following challenge.

'The pragmatic, reductionist stance which has come to dominate the ADHD field in the United States, while representing one range of beliefs, interpretations and mandates for action, does not necessarily translate well into many American sub-cultures, or cultures and societies outside the United States. The implicit assumptions held by any society, its professions and policymakers come under scrutiny at the intellectual, cultural and geographic borders. Thus, each society interested in ADHD as a category of mental disorder must first deal with the inherent cultural foundations which have been rendered invisible in the American field.'

Dr Katherine Ideus, US ADHD researcher

Does social class count?

While studies suggest drug use for ADHD is an upper middle-class trend in the US, it's different in Australia. Research of this type has not been conducted in New Zealand; it would provide a fascinating comparison. However, in my research in Australia there appear to be clusters of children using medication in both low-income areas and upper middle-class areas – though their reasons for taking drugs seem to be very different.

In my experience, most young people with ADHD are diagnosed at one of two ages. The first is between seven and nine years, and usually because of hyperactive behaviours in primary school. The second is 13 and 14 years, and usually because of inattention. At first, I thought that those diagnosed in their teens had either passed unnoticed through primary school or found ways to compensate because they were gifted. But as I explored the students' stories further, once I had accounted for the differences in diagnostic type by gender, it seemed that a child's diagnosis was more closely linked to socioeconomics than actual behaviour or difficulty at school. The students from the upper middle-class area tended to be diagnosed with the inattentive sub-type while those from lower-income areas were diagnosed with the hyperactive/impulsive sub-type. In other words, in my research if you lived in a low-income area you were more likely to be diagnosed in mid-primary school as 'hyperactive', while if you were middle class you were more likely to be diagnosed 'inattentive' in early secondary school.

With more competition at school and work, the use of ADHD drugs for children in Australia, New Zealand and America can be a tool to improve performance. There is a lot of pressure on our young people and many cannot afford to be just 'normal' if they are to reach the levels of success that they and their parents aspire to. This is not only because competition for the best university courses is tough, but also because many employers now expect higher standards of education for both apprenticeships and jobs that once required little senior secondary education.

With these demands on children to work harder, parents who are juggling family and long working hours may not have the time to give the support they would like to with homework and research. While some children can manage the pressure, those with ADHD are less likely to cope so well. Not surprisingly, many parents – believing that private education provides better education and individual support – spend a great deal to send their children to private schools, and when they don't do well, the parents look for reasons why. ADHD may be attractive to some upper middle-class parents because they see ADHD as both an explanation for why their child is not at the top of the class as well as a way of turning things around.

There's also the possibility that children from different social backgrounds may be judged differently. In one US study, researcher Gwendolyn Stevens got different groups of teachers to look at identical videotapes of children. Some groups were given summaries that described the children in the videos as middle class, others were given summaries describing the children as from low-income families. The result? Teachers rated the children described as from low-income families as being more hyperactive.

Remember too that when children from disadvantaged areas start school, they're going into a public education system where values tend to be middle class – so it's not surprising that social cues, ways of communicating and rules for disci-

> If you lived in a low-income area you were more likely to be diagnosed as 'hyperactive', while if you were middle class you were more likely to be diagnosed 'inattentive'

pline in these schools are more likely to mirror what middle-class kids are used to even before they put on a school uniform. This means that children from lower-income areas who may have been brought up with different rules and expectations are often disadvantaged from day one.

While some children adjust, others may feel frustrated and marginalised – and if this leads to disruptive behaviour, then it's likely to be the children (not the system) that get the blame. Making things even harder is the fact that these children may also have parents who lack the confidence or knowledge to get support for their child at school. It's into this scenario that the ADHD label appears, with its free visits to a medical practitioner and subsidised drug treatment for poorer families, as well as the potential to justify more school support.

Let's for a moment consider the story of Lionel, a 14-year-old participant in my research. Although it's a few years since I first met Lionel, his story and the emotion with which he told it is still clearly fixed in my mind.

The first thing you noticed about Lionel was the dirty, red basketball cap that never left his head, and the two ice-blue eyes gazing out from underneath it. He went to a poorly-funded government school in a low-income area and always seemed a little amazed by the world. He was a gentle and considerate kid, and it often seemed that the harsh environment that he found himself in whirred by so fast he was just carried along like a bit of driftwood. While the other students seemed to have some control over their lives, Lionel often seemed vague and at a loss. I worried about his future.

On one occasion, I asked him directly: 'What about your family Lionel, who's there and what do they do?'

'I've got a real dad and a stepdad ... I live with my real mum and stepdad ... cause my other dad is up north ... I don't give a shit where ...'

'Did he clear out then?'

'Yeah, he didn't care about me, I don't care either ...'. Lionel paused. 'And I've got a big brother who's 17 and my real dad tried to take him away from us, but we got him back and it went through the court and that ... yeah.'

Another pause. 'What about your stepdad?' I asked.

'He's unemployed, he doesn't work. On the dole I think, and umm, my mum works at a primary school, cleaning ... and my brother used to be a chef, but his boss got in another chef and wouldn't give him his pay cheque, and he got pissed off like ... and she finally gave him his cheque and it was only for $110 ...'

'Okay,' I said, 'and how long have you been at this school?'

'Just this year,' he replied cautiously.

Our conversation continued for a few minutes until Lionel came around to talking about ADHD and his medication. 'They've been trying me on dex to help me at school, but it stuffs me around. Like if I'm off it, I can't stay in my seat and get in heaps of trouble, but if I take it, I get really relaxed ... like I forget stuff and teachers ask me questions and I can't understand them. Like on my medication I forget stuff, and when I'm off it I can't sit still, I'm stuffed either way. They said I might be repeating Year Eight. I don't want to, I'm doin' my best, I want to go up.'

Lionel stopped speaking. There were tears in his eyes.

It's hard to know why ADHD diagnosis seems more of a middle-class phenomenon in the US, while in Australia it's in both low-income and upper middle-class families. It may be that in the Antipodes there's a broader spread of Anglo-Saxons across class lines, but before we can make this claim, research in New Zealand is required. Meanwhile, in upper middle-class areas it seems that ADHD is about treating inattention and boosting success at school; in lower-income areas it's more about controlling hyperactivity and keeping students in the classroom. This said, the link between ADHD and social class needs more research – perhaps it will find that an ADHD diagnosis is a way of taming the behaviour of children who feel that the rest of society is neglecting them. Or perhaps it is something more affluent families use to make sure their children succeed, and that poorer families use to make sure their kids don't miss out altogether? Much more research is needed if we are to adequately answer this question.

ADHD overseas

There are good reasons why ADHD seems to be more common in affluent Western nations. Medical services and record-keeping tend to be more efficient in these countries, so it's easier to keep track of patterns of health problems. Meanwhile, for poorer countries battling to meet the population's basic needs for health, nutrition and education, issues like behaviour problems aren't priorities. Better education and access to information in wealthier countries also means families are more aware of ADHD, and more affluence means more resources to help children with the disorder.

With so little data available on ADHD in many parts of the world, there have been few international comparisons of the disorder. However, in the mid-1990s the British Psychological Society estimated that ADHD affected less that one percent of children in the UK, while Australia and the US had estimated rates of between two and five percent. Although rates have increased more recently in New Zealand and Canada to match these levels, no industrialised nations in Europe or Asia have had such a dramatic growth in drug use to treat behavioural difficulties in children as Australia and the US. In Europe, diagnosis and drug use for ADHD is significantly lower in the UK, Spain and Holland, and it is very low in France, Denmark and Sweden. However, European ADHD websites are beginning to appear and interest is growing in France, but even when ADHD is identified, other approaches are still used first, with medication used only if other measures don't work. In Africa, the growing prominence of ADHD in American media and on the Internet is resulting in early signs of a growing awareness and diagnosis in South Africa and Zimbabwe. In Asia, there is some early – but very early – research beginning to identify ADHD in India, but otherwise ADHD is virtually unknown, a situation mirrored in South America.

Until recently, most studies comparing Australia and the US to other countries argued that the higher levels of ADHD in those countries were due to different methods of diagnosis. The country used to highlight this comparison was usually the UK, which uses the World Health Organisation's *ICD-10* (see Appendix A), rather than the American Psychiatric Association's *DSM-IV* (see Chapter 2). Compared to the *DSM-IV*, behaviour needs to be more extreme to be diagnosed as ADHD under the *ICD-10*, which may mean fewer children are diagnosed with ADHD under the WHO checklist. But this alone cannot account for variations in diagnosis, and as Professor Paul Cooper of Cambridge University points out, levels are lower in the UK because it has a history of social rather than medical approaches to emotional and behavioural problems.

In some countries, ADHD diagnosis varies not just by gender, ethnic background and social class, but also from one region to another. In both the US and Australia – which both use the same checklist to diagnose the disorder – there are variations according to where you live. So if ADHD is an evenly distributed genetic condition and diagnostic checklists are objective and accurate, how do you explain these variations? With widespread media coverage of ADHD in Australia and the US, it's unlikely that there's less awareness of the disorder in some areas, so there must be other factors.

One view is that the influence of American popular culture may be a factor. Australian television is swamped with American-based or -influenced content, and it would be naïve to think that this does not influence how young people see themselves and the world. ADHD is now an established part of American popular culture, and regularly appears in television and music media. The moment that Bart Simpson was labelled with ADHD on 'The Simpsons' was the confirmation that the disorder had shifted out of the medical textbooks and into the public mind. The archetype of Bart has even been adopted for academic research, with a recent University of Western Australia study using Bart to test student and parent perceptions of ADHD behaviours and their caricatures.

Despite this, it would be ambitious to think that American popular culture alone explains the growth of ADHD in Australia and New Zealand, because other countries (equally exposed to American cultural influence) have not followed US trends with ADHD. Is it that other nations and cultures are more resilient to American pop culture, or is there another explanation?

I don't believe there's any one simple explanation as to why Australasia and North America have higher rates of drug use. If I have a fear, it's that we have blindly followed US trends –

including the emphasis on ADHD as a purely medical problem – because of the strong influence of US culture at a time of globalisation and confusion over cultural identity. To see how real this fear is, I will now look at the example of the global and national pressures influencing ADHD in Australia.

Social change and ADHD in Australia

Although it has been discussed in previous chapters, it is important to reinforce the link between the growth in drug use for ADHD and recent social pressures in Australia. Some experts believe ADHD is the result of a mismatch between what a person is capable of and what contemporary society expects of them – in other words, ADHD may be a normal human response to the challenges of a society that's changed so fast that not everyone can keep up. Others even suggest that what's different about children with ADHD is that they haven't lost some of the traits that were so useful to our hunter-gatherer ancestors. Rather, these qualities, once essential to survival, are now at odds with current social standards. To hunter-gatherers, being impulsive and energetic helped you stay alive – faced with a hungry predator, you wouldn't spend too much time thinking about what to do next.

While some health professionals argue that medication use is a practical and humane way to help children meet social expectations and cope in their environment, some sociologists suggest that treating ADHD this way can be seen as a kind of social control – a way of weeding out difficult behaviour in a society and preserving conformity. Or, to put it another way, instead of trying to create a fairer society, using a label like ADHD helps cover up the shortcomings of a competitive society that lets many children down – and neatly shifts the blame back on to their bodies and their families.

Whatever your view, the world in which so many children are now diagnosed with ADHD has changed immensely in the last 30 years. Life moves faster, working hours are longer. According to the Australia Institute, Australians now work longer hours than the Germans, the Americans, and even the Japanese, and our competitive workplace now wants employees who are not only smart and creative, but focused and compliant as well. This means schools now have the job of trying to instil these conflicting qualities in their students to make them workplace-ready. Some young people can cope with this, but with such huge social and technological shifts in such a short time, it's a big ask to expect all human beings – diverse as they are – to adapt to these new rules in less than one generation. This is why it's worth considering ADHD as a product of social change. Look at it this way, and you begin to see ADHD as a problem partly created by our society's values. You begin to ask just who is failing whom and how fair and desirable are these priorities for Australia's future?

A label like ADHD helps cover up the shortcomings of a competitive society that lets many children down – and neatly shifts the blame back on to their bodies and their families

Pondering this question leads one to start looking at the big social changes that have occurred at the same time as the growth of ADHD. For instance, over the last 20 years all Western countries have felt the effects of globalisation. Pressures to keep a competitive edge in a global market and build a firm economic base for the future have tested all Western economies. For the most part Australia has tended to follow US and British policies of encouraging competition and reducing government interference in the economy. This has meant it's increasingly up to individuals to make up for any problems they have, rather than counting on the support of the government. The mantra that we all now recognise is the needy's responsibility to the taxpayer, rather than the taxpayer's responsibility to the needy.

In Australia, the result has been more responsibility placed on families to provide a safety net for their child. In this context, if you're a parent trying to get the best for your child with difficulty, anything that offers more help is welcome. For some families, a diagnosis of ADHD can be seen as a way of getting support at a time when there is more interest in investing in the economy than in investing in welfare to the community.

Not that this emphasis on nurturing the economy is all bad. The standard of living and affluence of Australians has grown dramatically over the last 50 years, and many families of children with ADHD have benefited from this change – although the growing gap between rich and poor in Australia also means others may not be doing so well. However, as the majority of Australia has become better off, it's also become increasingly urbanised and overworked. One result of this has been less time for family life and for involvement in traditional community networks.

In the past, we had to rely on the communities around us to help us survive. However, increasing affluence and the rise of technology have made us more independent – we don't need to rely on each other as much. While we haven't lost the commitment to others in our national psyche (which shows itself at times of crisis, like bushfire or drought), our daily lives are becoming more self-sufficient and anonymous, and our need for community is more likely to be met through television or Internet discussion groups. It is questionable whether these virtual communities can provide the safety net that families and communities once provided together.

When I was growing up in regional South Australia, people knew me, they knew my parents, and I knew I was accountable for my actions. My parents may not have been supervising me all the time, but I had a place and a responsibility. Yet many young people today don't have these networks or accountability to the same extent. With families more fragmented, there may not be strong links with grandparents; with busier work lives there may not be time to foster family friendships and other positive role-modelling relationships. Often we do not know the name of the person across the street, and for our kids this can leave them cut loose and without a broader accountability network.

Also, with both parents already working to support the high costs of a home, a car and a holiday, any extra expenses to support their children's needs add more pressure. Young people with emotional and behavioural needs often benefit from having adults in their lives who act as good role models – but this leaves hard-pressed parents between a rock and a hard place: they need to be available for their children, but they also need to work to support them (possibly working overtime to pay for any professional help they might need). Just to add to the pressure, children with emotional and behavioural difficulties don't cope well with the kind of stress that this situation can create in a family, nor with the lack of structure that goes with coming home to an empty house.

While none of these social changes cause ADHD, they do help to explain why families find relief in the disorder being diagnosed. When families are doing their utmost, but their best never seems to be enough, ADHD helps them make sense of what's going on and helps them cope. Yet this is a problem that shouldn't be shouldered by families alone. As a community we need to provide more support for vulnerable young people – where once they had a place, an identity and felt part of the community, now they're often left floundering. Also, we need to think about what we can do as leaders, community members or neighbours to ensure that the inevitable social changes of modern life benefit us all.

With all these things moving swiftly forward, we are faced with a complex situation if we want to help young people with ADHD. At times it seems all too much, and simple answers can be very attractive, but a tendency to oversimplify difficult issues doesn't help families living with ADHD. We have a bad habit of taking a problem out of its complex context, reducing it to a single issue and finding a single solution. In the case of nutrition, it's blaming our bad diets and finding solutions in vitamin pills. In the case of mental health, it's blaming depression and seeking drug therapy. And with behavioural problems, it's reducing the cause to some deficit in the individual that can be treated with amphetamines. The danger of this reductionist approach is that it ignores *all* the influences on human beings.

Traditionally a nation of down-to-earth pragmatists, it is perhaps not surprising that Australians have embraced a social philosophy that says because society is too big and too complex, we should focus just on helping the individual. This is especially the case when this view is reinforced by a preference for quick fixes in popular culture and the media. So when families are faced with high youth unemployment and growing competition in schools, you can understand the appeal of quick, pragmatic interventions. In the life of children, months or even weeks can be crucial to their development. In this situation, ADHD provides a practical solution – even if it involves drugs.

But then again it may be that Australian culture has been deeply medicalised since the 1950s, in a trend that's seen more and more life stages defined as illnesses – and the idea that we can find solutions to problems in pills. In my work as a secondary teacher at a predominantly white, middle-class school, not a day went by when a student didn't need to go to the front office or sick room for paracetamol. Given that there are other equally legitimate reasons or excuses for leaving the classroom, I wonder if it's a reflection of this medicalisation. In Australian popular culture, there's a belief that alleviating the pain is alleviating the problem, which makes many families and their children prime targets for using drugs to treat problematic life stages. This thinking shows up in this quote from recent research by Dr Georgia Carragher on Western Australian adolescents with ADHD:

'ADD is just like having a headache and you take Panadol or something like that and it gets rid of it, it doesn't get rid of it straight away, but it gets rid of it.'

The rejection of difference

Another trend that may influence ADHD is the changes in Australian cultural identity and attitudes toward difference. The white, British identity that dominated Australian society since the eighteenth century began changing in the 1980s and early 1990s when Australian governments did more to embrace ethnic and indigenous communities. But since the return of a conservative government – and possibly September 11 and the 2002 Bali bombings too – all this has waned. Instead, we have a renewed emphasis on more traditional notions of identity and behaviour. This presents a problem for young boys if we go back to promoting the Anzac ideal (which, along with courage and having a go, also includes being rebellious, energetic and anti-authoritarian). If we are encouraging them to model the qualities that helped the Anzacs, bushrangers and early pioneers to survive, but at the same time expecting people to be passive and compliant, aren't we sending mixed messages? In the case of ADHD, could it be that these changing attitudes see us medicate children with one hand in order to pacify the behaviours we encourage with the other?

As there is a shift away from a multicultural embrace of cultural diversity – at least for now – Australians are less clear about who they are, what they want and what their cultural priorities should be. This shaky cultural base, along with a retreat to right-wing conservative cultural values, leaves Australia vulnerable to a wave of similar values from the American context. Could it be that our inability to settle on a new cultural identity that accepts our diversity is one reason why we have not been as resilient as other nations? Is this why we have yet to respond to Ideus's challenge to come up with a way of coping with ADHD that reflects our own cultural experience?

Australians and New Zealanders are often surprised to learn that ADHD is largely an Australasian and North American phenomenon. Much of this surprise comes from the belief that has been perpetuated: that ADHD is a scientifically-endorsed category with conclusive medical tests. Yet the differences in rates of ADHD and drug treatment between many countries must be due to more than just different diagnostic practices. Global, national and cultural influences clearly play a part in who's identified, diagnosed and treated for ADHD. That Australia and New Zealand have followed US trends tells us more about recent cultural priorities than it does about improved medical practice.

ADHD is a real need in our society, but it's a need that is shaped by the surrounding culture and society. In this chapter, I've considered how ethnicity, economies, class and culture have all influenced ADHD. Rarely has ADHD been considered in such a way, and it leads to a new challenge for politicians, researchers and the community: while the ADHD label is our best way of understanding the challenges facing young people now, is it the best way of meeting their needs in the future? Are we producing a situation where more people need disorders like ADHD just to fit into society?

Key points

- If you are male, white and from a lower-income area, you are more likely to be diagnosed ADHD and treated with drugs.

- It seems a little hypocritical to embrace a national identity that praises the anti-authoritarian, impulsive and energetic qualities of the Anzacs, but then drug these qualities out of our kids.

- That Australia has followed the US in ADHD trends tells us more about social changes than about new medical theories or practice.

- One of these important changes is the growing acceptance of medical treatments for social problems.

- We should not only be asking how our kids with ADHD are failing society, but also how our society is failing our kids.

8

ADHD and politics

'I think we're seeing incredible increases in children who are just not able to cope with the education system. We're seeing an epidemic of four-, five-, six- and seven-year-olds with behaviour problems. In the developed world on the whole, about one in five teenagers has a significant mental illness ... if you look at all of the sorts of things that are pathways to mental ill health and to suicide, every single one of those pathways has actually been increasing. And at the same time, a lot of services for children have actually been stopped or underfunded.'

Professor Fiona Stanley, 2003 Australian of the Year

Professor Fiona Stanley is a paediatrician and director of the Telethon Institute for Child Health Research in Western Australia. She's one of many health professionals sounding alarm bells about the growing number of children and young people with psychosocial problems. She too – as I argued in the last chapter – believes that the rise in problems with mental health, learning disabilities, ADHD and other behavioural problems is more than just the sum of each individual situation. Professor Stanley advocates a preventative approach sometimes known as the 'fence at the top of the cliff'. It means you find a way to stop people hurting themselves because it's smarter than the alternative approach: parking the ambulance at the bottom of the cliff to cart the injured off to hospital. If we want to improve our children's mental health and grow healthy future generations of Australians, she says governments must put children first, by:

- boosting support structures for families;
- providing more funding so that children with potential problems can be identified and treated early; and
- looking at which government policies could be having a negative impact on families.

Such proposals put politicians firmly in the spotlight and can make governments nervous, and not just about the cost. One reason why it's hard to get governments to pay for preventative programs is that it's not always easy to measure how successful they will be. If we bring in programs to prevent future problems, how can we tell how many children would have had problems – or fallen off the cliff – if the programs hadn't been there? How do politicians justify this spending to the electorate? It's much easier to count how many bandages were used than how many accidents never occurred. But as Fiona Stanley warns, if we don't pay the cost of preventing problems, the cost of treating mental illness and behavioural disorders will have a real impact on Australian society in the future. It is a warning echoed by the National Health and Medical Research Council Report into ADHD as well as other Australian research.

'ADHD is having a wide impact in Australia. Disruptive behaviour at home produces high levels of stress in parents and children, sometimes stretching relationships to breaking point. Pressure is placed on teachers to maintain discipline and facilitate learning despite the academic difficulties often associated with ADHD. School administrators are expected to provide adequate resources for teachers at a time when real-term funding for government schools is declining. A range of health professionals (including doctors and psychologists) is approached with the expectation that they can make these children "normal". Politicians are lobbied to provide resources for counselling and support agencies for families, and for subsidised medication and disability allowances.'

I. M. Atkinson, J. A. Robinson and R. Shute

Yet when I ask young people about the role of politics in ADHD, they're usually either mystified or cynical.

'What've politicians got to do with ADD? They wouldn't care anyway.'

Daniel, 12 years

Such remarks aren't surprising. When you have a label that says your brain chemistry causes you problems, and you live with the daily heartache of difficulties with relationships, it can be hard to see how the bigger picture affects your situation. Yet ADHD has grown rapidly into a political issue.

ADHD – the political hot potato

What is making ADHD hard to handle is that there is currently no official policy dedicated to it at either State or Federal level.

Responsibility for services belongs to State governments because they're largely responsible for delivering health and education services. Following legal advice, the States have avoided developing specific ADHD policy out of concerns that it might open a floodgate of claims and leave them liable. Consequently, State governments claim there's no need for a specific ADHD policy because the needs of children with ADHD are already being met under existing policies and with existing services. And the Commonwealth Government has seen no need to intervene with the States.

What is making ADHD hard to handle is that there is currently no official policy dedicated to it at either State or Federal level

But there is much more behind the reluctance of governments to develop policy on ADHD than merely concerns about who should pay for services:

- In addition to government fear of opening the floodgates of eligibility, there are also concerns over misdiagnosis and the possibility of children who don't have the disorder using up already limited resources.

- The diverse nature of the challenges associated with ADHD crosses many different State and Federal departments. For instance, should the disorder be an education, health, disability, justice or welfare issue? With something as complex and controversial as ADHD, it's no surprise to hear some ministers explain that it's the responsibility of another department.

- Also, the growing investment of governments in media units and political advertising has perpetuated a 'one-term outlook' and an emphasis on projects that get results within three to four years. Complex issues like ADHD require a long-term strategy, and can linger on the back-burner because of a reluctance to be seen to fail in the short term or to invest in a long-term project for which your party may not receive the credit.

- There are also issues about promoting any policy or initiatives to the voting public. ADHD has become so controversial that few politicians or parties with an eye on government at the next election are prepared to take on something so risky.

Whatever the reasons for the lack of proactive political response to ADHD, the realm of politics has not been without its effect. There's little doubt in my mind that the lack of proactive political responses to ADHD in Australia has contributed to the growth in drug use to treat the disorder.

Recent Australian political history and ADHD

To understand the impact of Australian politics on ADHD, it's important to put the current situation in a historical context. To do this, let's return to post-war Australia and chart its journey toward the globalisation that saw ADHD land on our shores.

After the trauma of the Depression and World War Two, Australians backed the idea that everyone had the right to work and to have access to adequate welfare services. The Federal Government expanded the welfare state, putting services like electricity, gas and transport under state ownership and making reforms in housing and education. All this was affordable because there was a healthy demand overseas for Australian agricultural and mineral products, and manufacturing industries were protected with high tariffs.

In the 1950s and 1960s, we saw a long era of conservative rule in Australia. Under Prime Minister Menzies, the Australian economy shifted away from government control and toward more private enterprise, only to be changed again in the early 1970s, when many Australians voted in a young and idealistic Labor government. The leadership of Gough Whitlam brought a wide range of social reforms, including a national health scheme and more funding to education. These changes saw health and education elevated to national concerns, and aimed to create greater equality by using the Federal Government's greater revenue-raising capacity. However, the cost of implementing them came at a time when the Australian economy ran into trouble.

The resulting financial problems brought a dramatic and lasting change to Australia's economic thinking. From the time of Whitlam, the attitude to Asian countries changed: instead of seeing them as potential invaders, we increasingly saw the need to be trading with them. It was this new view that was vital to Australia's entry into the global economy and behind the Hawke and Keating governments forging closer economic ties with Asia (which have been continued under the current Howard government).

But as Australia entered international markets, it exposed itself to the dramatic economic changes that were going on internationally. The nature of work as we'd known it began to change, with a decline in old-style manufacturing and many low-skilled jobs, and more

While affluent families can afford private health insurance and the range of therapies to give children multi-modal treatment, poorer families struggle to make ends meet

demand for workers educated in information technology. And while globalisation has helped Australia boost its economic strength, the emphasis on boosting productivity, efficiency and profits has had its downside. By following a philosophy of economic rationalism to cut government spending, Federal and State governments alike have reduced their involvement in providing health, welfare and education services by shifting responsibility for them to the private sector. The idea behind this is that private companies do things more efficiently (i.e., in a more cost-effective way) than the public service. Governments also now encourage a greater role for charities to provide health and welfare services, and even for companies to provide corporate sponsorship of community services.

Linked to this is government rhetoric about how people receiving assistance have an obligation to the taxpayer – instead of the taxpaying community having a responsibility to those in need. There's also the attitude among neo-liberal governments that many problems like ADHD are not so much public health issues as deficiencies within individuals – as a result, it's up to them, their families, or non-government services to provide support. Such an approach has no problem with cuts to funding or to redefining criteria for eligibility to reduce the number of families relying on government support. A good example of how this works can be seen in a comment made by Labor Senator for WA, Mark Bishop, in 2003:

> *'The Minister cannot escape the fact that the new child disability assessment tool was designed to further restrict access to this payment. To justify these cuts ... she makes the assertion that many children who have lost the allowance have somehow outgrown their disability. This may be the case in some instances ... but she ignores the many families who through hard work and medical advice learn to better manage disabilities. Some examples that come to mind are chronic asthma, diabetes, ADD and ADHD – to name but a few. The fact is that conditions such as these involve considerable time and costs. Many are only under control because of the expensive treatment that the carer allowance assists with.'*

Meanwhile, the traditional protectors of people in need – left-wing thinkers and politicians – are struggling to mount an argument that can catch the public's imagination. While the right hand of politics has developed an everyday philosophy based on working hard and looking out for yourself, the left has been unable to convince most Australians that because there is no level playing field, the argument that the hardworking will prosper makes little sense. Neither have they been able to convince governments of the need to protect funding to education, health and welfare so that no-one misses out. Instead, spending on education in Australia has been just over 4.5 percent of GDP (the measure of national wealth) for 2000–2005, compared to 6.7 percent of GDP in 1975. What we are putting into education has fallen well below the average for OECD countries, and many Australians have felt the pinch of these changes. As the resulting gap between rich and poor grows, and there is less public sector support for special needs in real terms, the notion that Australia was built on 'a fair go' through full employment and welfare sounds more and more nostalgic.

So what have these recent big-picture political changes meant for ADHD? In the case of health and welfare under neo-liberal politics, it's increasingly up to families to pay for services for children with ADHD. As governments reduce their involvement in health services to encourage more private health insurance, the responsibility for non-drug treatment of ADHD is shifting to private health professionals. While affluent families can afford private health insurance and the range of therapies to give children multi-modal treatment, poorer families struggle to make ends meet. For families with a health care card, Medicare provides access to certain medical practices through bulk-billing, and the Pharmaceutical Benefits Scheme allows affordable access to dexamphetamine (and methylphenidate, as of August 2005). In contrast, waiting lists for government services providing non-drug therapies that children and families with ADHD may need (such as speech therapy, remedial education, social skills development or family therapy) have been up to two years. In terms of a child's development, this is a long time, and many parents may give up trying to access multi-modal treatment through government services.

'When my son was three his speech was unintelligible – the
waiting list for speech therapy services through the hospital
was a year, so we had to see a private speech therapist. It
cost me $90 a week.'

Single mother of a boy with ADHD

But what if you cannot afford $90 a week for treatment? While
governments claim that multi-modal treatment is available, the
reality is that families can't always wait for as long as it takes to
access them. This may help explain the higher use of drugs to
treat ADHD in less affluent parts of Australia. For instance, if
you're on a low income and your choices are either waiting a
year to access service, or paying a fee for a private service, or
else an appointment with a doctor (who may prescribe affordable medication) in two weeks' time, it's obvious which will be
the choice of many families. In the absence of adequate policy
and resourcing, drugs cease to be the last resort and become the
only resort for these families.

School principals and educational researchers back up the
complaints that parents make about inadequate services. In
basic terms, funding to public education hasn't kept pace with
inflation in recent years, and although this has affected all
schools, the impact has been more dramatic in areas where
less affluent schools and higher numbers of children with ADHD
collide.

'Students who are depressed, suffering eating disorders,
involved in substance abuse, living in stressful family
settings, embarking on a pattern of offending, engaged in
chronic truanting or who have difficulties managing
conflict are, according to school principals, much less
likely to be rapidly attended to than they would have been
five or six years previously. Such delays are difficult for the

*young people and place considerable strain on their
families, friends and teachers.'*

Professor Pat Thomson, former principal in
Adelaide's urban fringe

Disadvantaged schools in places like the northern suburbs of
Adelaide (a region of high ADHD treatment with medication)
report a significant deterioration in access to the kinds of health
services that make a difference – general and mental health services, welfare services, community policing. This is a direct result
of decisions to cut funds to these services. But what of the claims
of governments that these needs are being met under other
existing policies?

ADHD and policy – how kids fall through the cracks

As mentioned earlier in the chapter, the responsibility for ADHD
currently rests with State governments, and there's no official
policy dedicated to the problem at either State or Commonwealth
level. Each State has different legislation on ADHD, but these laws
mostly relate to medication use. While equal opportunity laws
recognise equality of access to services, in reality this isn't much
help because the Education Department guidelines that are
based on this equal opportunity legislation don't specify any tan-
gible resource support for children with ADHD. Instead, they
spell out the range of educational strategies teachers should use
with all kids and outline existing services for children with
particular needs. This means it's up to schools and individual
teachers to find the best way of helping children with ADHD –
but without the back-up of extra time or resources to help them.

The level of support that children with ADHD can expect
from State education departments varies from State to State, and
often from school to school, but what all States have in common

is that instead of identifying problems early on (the 'fence at the top of the cliff' approach), you have to wait for a crisis before treatment becomes available. This is the total opposite of what's considered the best treatment practice for ADHD (i.e. getting in as early as possible with whatever educational or psychosocial support, or other services, a child needs). So how do departments justify their position?

Most State Education Department guidelines argue that labels are harmful and that although ADHD is an educational risk factor, it's not in itself grounds for extra help or a specific policy. In Western Australia, however, a 1999 parliamentary inquiry into ADHD found that a significant barrier to the effective treatment of ADHD was the fact that education departments treated ADHD as one of many disorders that may place a child at educational risk, rather than as a separate learning and behaviour category. It recommended that the State Government develop new policies and guidelines for ADHD. This response is an exception, but if it were to become the basis of policy, the US 'Child Find' system would need to be looked at closely. Under that system, any organisation that receives Federal funding – schools, for example – must check for children with disorders and make sure they have the treatment they need. This shifts the responsibility from parents to prove their child has a problem, and onto the school to make an assessment and intervene. If this approach was introduced in Australia, it could potentially reduce the number of families who use medication simply because it's the only treatment they can access. Not surprisingly, some politicians have already called for changes that would introduce a 'Child Find' clause and encourage earlier treatment, but the response from governments so far is that it's too expensive.

So, although existing policy theoretically covers all students with special needs, in practice only those with extreme difficulties receive help, and often ADHD doesn't get high priority. In some States, students need to be more than five years behind in their literacy and numeracy development, or have had a history of expulsion before they get priority for limited resources. In many States it was once the case that students received help when they fell two years behind, but now lack of resources have changed policies to four years – which in practice is more than five once they pass through referral and other waiting lists.

Another explanation of why the needs of so many children with ADHD aren't met is that there can be a gap between what government departments recommend and how these recommendations are put into practice. In short, policy documents are like a tool: how they're used can depend on the knowledge and skill of who's using them. A doctor who's interpreting a policy, for instance, is more likely to see ADHD from the point of view of medical research, while a counsellor may be more influenced by popular opinion. This can potentially create a scenario where one professional prescribes drugs while the other dismisses a child's needs as bad behaviour. Even within a profession, such as teaching, there can be a great difference between the intention of guidelines, how teachers interpret them, and what it looks like in the classroom. In other words, the same policies may be interpreted and used very differently – especially when you have no specific ADHD policy.

> **It's up to schools and individual teachers to find the best way of helping children with ADHD – but without the back-up of extra time or resources to help them**

From my experience working as an advisor in state politics, it seems that ADHD has proven too hot to handle for both major Australian political parties. In fact, my very entry into politics was shaped by the lack of response of the two major parties. After sending the findings and policy implications of my doctoral study to all political parties, it was only the Australian Democrats who responded to these findings. As a consequence, I came to be an advisor to that party on ADHD.

As both the Hon. Mike Elliott MLC (ex-South Australian Democrats leader) and the media pushed the then-Liberal Government in South Australia on the issue of ADHD, I watched its response with interest. As a matter of course, responsibility for ADHD was deferred to the medical profession, a position justified by the greater weight of research on ADHD from within that discipline. Unfortunately, such an argument does not take into account the greater funding available from pharmaceutical companies for medical research into ADHD and drug treatment, and the barriers to social research into ADHD over the last 40 years. What this produces is an imbalance of information and a potential (if unintentional) bias toward medical theories about ADHD (which, I have sought to argue in this book, is inadequate).

When questions emerged in parliament about the use of drugs for ADHD, the political response was invariably that there was no access to ADHD medication without the multi-modal treatment approach also being available. Without any reference to what might be happening in the community, the then-Liberal State Government argued that because this approach should be occurring, it *was* occurring, and there was no problem with ADHD. This ran contrary to ongoing concerns by those in non-medical professions working daily with ADHD, as well as to statistical studies showing large variations by region, income and numbers of prescribing doctors. It seemed that political responses were more about what needed to be true than what was actually occurring.

The usual pattern with these things is that a new study or media report prompts a more rigorous political response. Usually the Minister responsible would express concern and then announce a working party or inquiry to look into their concern. Using the example of my home state of South Australia, it has been in a constant state of inquiry since the mid-1990s, and at one time two inquiries were running simultaneously. Over this time, both Labor and Liberal have been in power, and numerous working-party and inquiry recommendations have been made, with little real action taken on them. The most recent inquiry (after significant delays in reporting) deferred its recommendations to a working group, which voted itself out of existence without addressing most of the inquiry's recommendations. Notably, the visionary recommendation for 'one-stop health shops' to enable access to multi-modal treatment (rather than medication treatment alone) has been left unaddressed. Meanwhile, a child diagnosed with ADHD at the age of seven when the inquiries started is now, in 2006, leaving school – and little has changed. While inquiries are often well-meaning, can reassure the public, and pacify the media, they can also be used as a political ploy to keep an issue static until it is no longer 'your problem'.

No doubt these comments will draw cries of 'unfair' from the parties involved, and a series of claims will be rolled out to dispel these accusations of inaction. But an important point remains: if past political responses to ADHD had worked effectively, one could expect that public and professional concerns about ADHD would have been addressed. Instead, drug use remains high, advocates are pushing ever harder for support, and teachers are more desperate than ever. No response to ADHD is in itself clearly a response, particularly at a time when governments are shifting a greater burden onto families to provide support. It is perhaps no surprise that there has been an increasing interest among ADHD advocates for the recognition of ADHD in existing disability policies.

ADHD a disability category?

ADHD cannot be properly understood without a consideration of the heated battle over resources. Parents seek out an ADHD diagnosis because they are unhappy with support from schools and other government agencies. However, after finding that diagnosis provides little additional support due to the limitations of the guidelines for special-needs assistance in schools, some families then try to have their child's needs recognised under the Commonwealth of Australia Disability Discrimination Act (or DDA, which recognises disorders listed by the *Diagnostic and Statistical Manual of Mental Disorders*, including ADHD). This means parents have to get their child assessed by a range of different health professionals – a process that takes time and money, with no guarantee of success.

> Gina, a mother of three children, told me she'd fought for three years to have her son's needs recognised by her State Government – a step that turned her into a fulltime advocate for ADHD. Even after her child was diagnosed with ADHD, she couldn't get support for him from the State Education Department. Gina wasn't well off, and had to decide the best way to use the money she had – either to pay for her son to have the therapies he needed, or use it to pay for assessments by specialists (and possibly qualify under the DDA). She opted to pay for the tests in the hope that it would help her son more in the long term – even though there was no guarantee that a favourable ruling would mean more support from the State Education Department. When we last spoke she was still battling, conscious that time and her son's opportunities at school were running out.

Most parents don't have the time or money for this. If children get non-drug treatments, it's usually because both parents work (often overtime) just to afford the range of professional services needed in multi-modal treatment. But for many poorer families, drugs may be the only affordable treatment – for them, qualifying under the DDA is an unrealistic dream.

One solution put forward has been to make ADHD an official learning disability category in State disability policy. The argument behind this is that it will ensure that student needs are met and supported with resources, but there are a few problems with this:

1   ADHD isn't a learning disability. While it may increase the chances of underachieving at school, it doesn't always lead to educational failure. Many children with ADHD are remarkably bright and their difficulties at school have as much to do other issues as they do with learning problems. These issues include a lack of skills (e.g. knowing how to write essays, how to take notes or how to construct an argument) as well as attitudes to success and behaviour at school. Some ADHD kids who are very bright use their ability to entertain the class and make smart remarks, rather than learn. Having ADHD doesn't inevitably make you dumb or bad at school.

2   Making ADHD a learning disability category is unlikely to provide extra educational support, especially when special education funding is already limited. Changing a name will make little difference if the money's not there; it just means more people will be competing for inadequate funds.

3   There's always the risk that calling ADHD a disability will just reinforce the idea that ADHD is a medical diagnosis, and imply that other approaches are less important.

So it's unlikely that making ADHD a learning disability will improve support, especially in the context of real-term funding cuts to education and disability services.

Making life easier

At the moment one can be excused for believing that life is so busy for most Australians that they do not have time for public debate on difficult issues, and instead hand over their taxes to pay politicians to make their public decisions for them. Possibly, with a Federal Government in control of both houses, controversial terrorism laws and industrial relations legislation, this may change, but for now it certainly seems the case. What this means for a complex problem like ADHD is that governments tread water: they manage the issue with as little involvement as possible until it can be delegated or handed over to the next minister or bureaucrat. This handling (or hand-passing) of the ADHD hot potato has helped drive 'medical-only' responses to ADHD and, I believe, has exacerbated the problems faced by families of children with the disorder. Not providing specific support has driven those in need elsewhere – to Medicare, the PBS and drug use. In the process, a medical model of ADHD has emerged by default which provides an imbalanced and inadequate understanding of ADHD.

Now is the time for public debate about ADHD. As parents, neighbours, teachers, community leaders and politicians, we need to look at the many faces of ADHD and not simply swallow the medical solution whole. Although life was not meant to be easy, surely life for families with ADHD was not meant to be this hard, and there are things that we can take to our politicians that can make life easier (in both the long and short term). In the remainder of this chapter I look at some of these.

How to clean up our act

1 Get a grip on drug use

The first challenge is drug use for ADHD. The United Nations has warned Australia about our high use of drugs to treat behaviour problems: Australia was the only nation other than the US that was identified for prescribing medication to children for behavioural disorders at concerning levels. Yet, just recently, the Commonwealth Government added Ritalin to the list of subsidised drugs in Australia, notably without any injection of funding for other, multi-modal treatments.

The higher rates of prescriptions for ADHD medication in some parts of Australia are also a concern. One way of discouraging over-prescription would be for the Federal

Government to introduce a system to make sure prescription rates are recorded consistently across the States, and highlight areas that may be above the national average. In these cases, public and political pressure should expose the cause of these higher rates.

2 *Tighten diagnosis and treatment*

Currently, there's no way of regulating how ADHD is diagnosed and treated. Although concerns about diagnostic practices a few years ago prompted a set of guidelines for doctors, none of them are actually enforceable with penalties. Although there have been times when concerns have been raised about some doctors' diagnostic practices, these have been dismissed by claims that the practitioner was doing research or was an expert in the field. If we had guidelines with penalties for practitioners who breach them, there'd be less confusion over diagnosis and more protection for both the public and the reputation of practitioners. This approach would mean State governments would have to:

- monitor the use of multi-modal treatment, as well as prescriptions, to see how widely they were being used;
- ensure restricted access to drugs until a multi-modal treatment plan had been registered. This would also ensure that drugs were being used as the last resort, not the first; and
- boost funding for non-medical support services to make multi-modal treatment more accessible.

3 *Improve government services*

Governments say services are available but families and teachers argue that long waiting lists make them hard to access. At the moment, there's no way of effectively testing either of these claims, and one advantage of monitoring all forms of treatment would be that we'd have a better idea of how widely multi-modal treatment is being used. The rapid rise in ADHD diagnosis and drug use alone questions official claims that multi-modal treatment is widely accessible. There also needs to be more teamwork between the different professionals involved in multi-modal treatment: one way forward could be to establish emotional and behavioural difficulty centres ('one-stop health shops') where a range of professionals are all at one site, and families can seek support or be referred by schools.

As has been highlighted, part of the problem is the gap between policy and practice in providing services for ADHD. The Federal Government needs to put more pressure on State governments to provide services by promoting a component similar to the American Child Find clause in the Disability Discrimination Act. In practice, this will mean all organisations and agencies who get federal funding will have to test for the needs of children under their care, rather than leaving it to families.

The Federal Government will also need to make the States close the gaps between the DDA and State equal opportunity legislation by defining a child's need as 'any barrier that stops them from having a productive life and getting a job'. On a practical level this would mean State governments would have to work harder to meet all the educational, behavioural and social needs of children. In schools, this could be done with an Individual Education Plan – a plan introduced at six years of age to identify and address a student's strengths and needs, and to be followed throughout a child's schooling. Besides helping all students, it would particularly help students with the complex set of needs that goes with ADHD.

4 Educate parents, the public and teachers

How about a national campaign to educate parents and the public about both sides of the disorder and the challenges of living with ADHD? A better-informed public would have more compassion for children with ADHD and would be more resilient to popular (mis)representations of ADHD from the US. A public campaign could include information to improve understanding of the social and biological aspects of the disorder, problems that cause similar behaviour and the range of support services available. Parents could receive better information on how to access services for their child. All these measures could help reduce diagnosis and drug use; and while they might be costly now, they'll prevent even greater costs later.

5 *Re-think our education priorities*

Federal and State governments also should look at how economic priorities in education are excluding more children who are entitled to fit into our society. We need to work out how to accommodate these children and give them meaningful pathways into adult life, rather than simply labelling them with a disorder and casting them loose. Given the Federal Government's interest in boys and schooling – in 2003 it held an inquiry into the needs of boys in school – the number of boys being excluded from school and labelled with ADHD should be a topic of some concern.

Professor Bob Lingard from the University of Sheffield, one of the authors of that Commonwealth inquiry, offers an interesting insight into the current economic pressure in education. He notes that as the current Federal Government has retreated from general and redistributive funding for education – at a time when the needs of those on the edge have increased with globalisation – we are now faced with an urgent need for new social justice policies that *include* rather than exclude. To do this, he says, we need to look closely at how factors such as class, gender, ethnicity and disability are coming together in complex ways to create new identities. When we understand these, politicians and policymakers can then form social justice policies that are targeted and equitable, and that help teachers to truly support those in need.

It is my view that ADHD represents one such coming-together of factors. It is an identity that needs to be understood, not just as a medical theory but as a social phenomenon. As such, it provides not only a window into contemporary Australian priorities but also an opportunity to move toward a more socially just society. It's a hot potato, but it's worth holding on to.

Key points

- The inadequacy of response to ADHD by politicians has contributed to the growth in drug use for ADHD in Australia.
- Many families are using drugs to treat ADHD either because it is the only treatment they know about or the only one they can afford.
- Early intervention for ADHD comes at a cost, but by waiting we face an even greater cost.
- ADHD is much more than a medical theory; it is an opportunity to explore policy for a more socially just society.

Epilogue:
A new view of ADHD

For many people, the links between ADHD and society seem all too abstract. They seem a world away from taking your kids to school each morning and hoping you don't get a crisis call during the day, or facing a classroom of 30 students and hoping you can find time to help the individuals with special needs. But right now we have one of three choices: we can try to change young people to fit modern society; we can try to change society to accept diversity; or we can give up, say it is all too hard and leave it to someone else.

Trying to pin responsibility for ADHD on a particular person, group or part of society has more to do with giving up than with tackling the issue. We need to recognise that ADHD is real because its consequences are real – and we need to share the responsibility of helping incorporate young people into a socially just society that accepts diversity through informed interactions, interventions and policy.

In this book I've argued that until recently, Australia, New Zealand and the US have largely stuck to making individuals fit into society and left it to medicine to provide the means for them to do so. The result is a situation where drug use has become attractive and convenient, placing minimal demand on everyone involved other than children with ADHD and their families.

Faced with the fact that the human gene pool cannot adapt at the rate that society has changed in the last 20 years, we have (perhaps inadvertently) relied on another technology, drugs, to control our young people. Under the guise of developing a practical and humane response to real need, there has emerged a lopsided view of ADHD. While medicine has given the impression of progress, little more than a Bandaid has been applied to a wound that cuts to the core values of our age. None of this is to diminish the good work being done by many dedicated professionals. Instead, it is to realise that ADHD is part of a dramatic change in our society during the last 20 years and that collectively we need to pause to contemplate how best to respond.

There's no neat solution to the human problem called ADHD. People have been, and will continue to be, biologically different, and the differences which society decides are problems will remain the product of their particular time and place in history. But if we don't start looking at ADHD as both a social and a medical condition, then in another 20 years we may still be facing the same problems, with the same limited solutions.

A new view of ADHD must recognise that the condition can vary according to the young person, their gender, ethnicity, social class and where they live. It can vary according to their environment, how other people respond to them, the media, political priorities and social values. A new view must avoid the one-size-fits-all approach that locates the problem in the individual, and look instead for a more holistic and socially just response.

In some way we're all responsible for ADHD because we promote, endorse, condone or ignore the values that exclude some but not others. We need a new, balanced approach to helping young people with ADHD. It is an approach that needs to value families and individual diversity, but also needs to acknowledge that the values we hold as a society can turn a difference into a problem. Only when we tackle how society is failing young people, will the labels that map out their failure become less relevant. For people who struggle with ADHD, it is such changes that offer the best way forward and in which our hopes reside.

Appendix A:
ADHD diagnostic criteria in Europe & the UK

In Chapter 2, I provided some details about the use of the APA's *DSM-IV* for diagnosis of ADHD in Australia and the US. Here is an extract from the WHO's *International Classification of Diseases*, which is used in Europe and the UK. You'll see that the WHO's terminology for the disorder that we call ADHD is different – it's known as 'hyperkinetic disorders'.

F90 Hyperkinetic disorders

This group of disorders is characterised by early onset; a combination of overactive, poorly modulated behaviour with marked inattention and lack of persistent task involvement; and pervasiveness over situations and persistence over time of these behavioural characteristics.

It is widely thought that constitutional abnormalities play a crucial role in the genesis of these disorders, but knowledge of specific etiology is lacking at present. In recent years, the use of the diagnostic term 'attention deficit disorder' for these syndromes has been promoted. It has not been used here because it implies a knowledge of psychological processes that is not yet available, and it suggests the inclusion of anxious, preoccupied, or 'dreamy' apathetic children whose problems are probably different. However, it is clear that, from the point of view of behaviour, problems of inattention constitute a central feature of these hyperkinetic syndromes.

Hyperkinetic disorders always arise early in development (usually in the first five years of life). Their chief characteristics are lack of persistence in activities that require cognitive involvement, and a tendency to move from one activity to another without completing any one, together with disorganised, ill-regulated, and excessive activity. These problems usually persist through school years and even into adult life, but many affected individuals show a gradual improvement in activity and attention.

Several other abnormalities may be associated with these disorders. Hyperkinetic children are often reckless and impulsive, prone to accidents, and find themselves in disciplinary trouble because of unthinking (rather than deliberately defiant) breaches of rules. Their relationships with adults are often socially uninhibited, with a lack of normal caution and reserve; they are unpopular with other children and may become isolated. Cognitive impairment is common, and specific delays in motor and language development are disproportionately frequent.

Secondary complications include unsocial behaviour and low self-esteem. There is accordingly considerable overlap between hyperkinesis and other patterns of disruptive behaviour such as 'unsocialised conduct disorder.' Nevertheless, current evidence favours the separation of a group in which hyperkinesis is the main problem.

Hyperkinetic disorders are several times more frequent in boys than in girls. Associated reading difficulties (and/or other scholastic problems) are common.

Diagnostic guidelines

The cardinal features are impaired attention and overactivity: both are necessary for the diagnosis and should be evident in more than one situation (e.g. home, classroom, clinic).

Impaired attention is manifested by prematurely breaking off from tasks and leaving activities unfinished. The children change frequently from one activity to another, seemingly losing interest in one task because they become diverted to another (although laboratory studies do not generally show an unusual degree of sensory or perceptual distractibility). These deficits in persistence and attention should be diagnosed only if they are excessive for the child's age and IQ.

Overactivity implies excessive restlessness, especially in situations requiring relative calm. It may, depending upon the situation, involve the child running and jumping around, getting up from a seat when he or she was supposed to remain seated, excessive talkativeness and noisiness, or fidgeting and wriggling. The standard for judgement should be that the activity is excessive in the context of what is expected in the situation and by comparison with other children of the same age and IQ. This behavioural feature is most evident in structured, organised situations that require a high degree of behavioural self-control.

The associated features are not sufficient for the diagnosis or even necessary, but help to sustain it. Lack of inhibition in social relationships, recklessness in situations involving some danger, and impulsive flouting of social rules (as shown by intruding on or interrupting others' activities, prematurely answering questions before they have been completed, or difficulty in waiting turns) are all characteristic of children with this disorder.

Learning disorders and motor clumsiness occur with undue frequency, and should be noted separately when present; they should not, however, be part of the actual diagnosis of hyperkinetic disorder.

Symptoms of conduct disorder are neither exclusion nor inclusion criteria for the main diagnosis, but their presence or absence constitutes the basis for the main subdivision of the disorder.

The characteristic behaviour problems should be of early onset (before age six years) and long duration. However, before the age of school entry, hyperactivity is difficult to recognise because of the wide normal variation: only extreme levels should lead to a diagnosis in preschool children.

Diagnosis of hyperkinetic disorder can still be made in adult life. The grounds are the same, but attention and activity must be judged with reference to developmentally appropriate norms. When hyperkinesis was present in childhood, but has disappeared and been succeeded by another condition, such as unsocial personality disorder or substance abuse, the current condition rather than the earlier one is coded.

Differential diagnosis

Mixed disorders are common, and pervasive developmental disorders take precedence when they are present. The major problems in diagnosis lie in differentiation from conduct disorder: when its criteria are met, hyperkinetic disorder is diagnosed with priority over conduct disorder. However, milder degrees of overactivity and inattention are common in conduct disorder. When features of both hyperactivity and conduct disorder are present, and the hyperactivity is pervasive and severe, 'hyperkinetic conduct disorder' (F90.1) should be the diagnosis.

A further problem stems from the fact that overactivity and inattention, of a rather different kind from that which is characteristic of a hyperkinetic disorder, may arise as a symptom of anxiety or depressive disorders. Thus, the restlessness that is typically part of an agitated depressive disorder should not lead to a diagnosis of a hyperkinetic disorder. Equally, the restlessness that is often part of severe anxiety should not lead to the diagnosis of a hyperkinetic disorder. If the criteria for one of the anxiety disorders are met, this should take precedence over hyperkinetic disorder unless there is evidence, apart from the restlessness associated with anxiety, for the additional presence of a hyperkinetic disorder. Similarly, if the criteria for a mood disorder are met, hyperkinetic disorder should not be diagnosed in addition simply because concentration is impaired and there is psychomotor agitation. The double diagnosis should be made only when symptoms that are not simply part of the mood disturbance clearly indicate the separate presence of a hyperkinetic disorder.

Acute onset of hyperactive behaviour in a child of school age is more probably due to some type of reactive disorder (psychogenic or organic), manic state, schizophrenia, or neurological disease (e.g. rheumatic fever).

Excludes:
* anxiety disorders
* mood (affective) disorders
* pervasive developmental disorders
* schizophrenia.

F90.0 Disturbance of activity and attention

There is continuing uncertainty over the most satisfactory subdivision of hyperkinetic disorders. However, follow-up studies show that the outcome in adolescence and adult life is much influenced by whether or not there is associated aggression, delinquency or unsocial behaviour. Accordingly, the main subdivision is made according to the presence or absence of these associated features. The code used should be F90.0 when the overall criteria for hyperkinetic disorder (F90.-) are met but those for conduct disorders are not.

Includes:
* attention deficit disorder or syndrome with hyperactivity
* attention deficit hyperactivity disorder.

Excludes:
* hyperkinetic disorder associated with conduct disorder (F90.1).

F90.1 Hyperkinetic conduct disorder

This coding should be used when both the overall criteria for hyperkinetic disorders (F90) and the overall criteria for conduct disorders are met.

Appendix B:
Further reading

Chapter 1 (An introduction to ADHD)

Russell A. Barkley (2006), *Attention Deficit Hyperactivity Disorder: A handbook for diagnosis and treatment*, 3rd Edition, Guilford Press: New York.

Lawrence Diller (2002), *Should I Medicate My Child?*, Basic Books: New York.

Chapter 2 (ADHD in Australia/NZ/UK)

Australia: National Health and Medical Research Council (1998), *Attention Deficit Hyperactivity Disorder*. Australian Government Publishing Service: Canberra.

NZ: Ministry of Health NZ (2001), *New Zealand Guidelines for the Assessment and Treatment of Attention Deficit / Hyperactivity Disorder,* NZ Ministry of Health: Wellington.

UK: British Psychological Society (1996), *Attention Deficit Hyperactivity Disorder (ADHD): a psychological response to an evolving concept,* Leicester: BPS.

Chapter 3 (The history of ADHD)

Kathy Baker (2004), *Reading Success: A reading intervention for students with ADHD*. Moorabbin, Victoria: Hawker Brownlow Education.

Peter Conrad (1976), *Identifying Hyperactive Children: the medicalization of deviant behaviour*, D.C. Heath & Co: USA.

Lawrence Diller (1998), *Running on Ritalin*, Bantam Books: New York.

R. Schachar (1986), 'Hyperkinetic Syndrome: historical development of the concept', in E. Taylor (ed.), *The Overactive Child*, Blackwell Publishers: Oxford, pp. 19–40.

Chapter 4 (Books to help you talk to young people about ADHD)

Biography: Ben Polis (2001), *Only a Mother Could Love Him*, Seaview Press: Adelaide.

Novel: Rosanne Hawke (2000), *The Keeper*, Lothian: Adelaide.

Play: Sean Riley (2005), *My Sister Violet*, Urban Myth Theatre: Adelaide.

Chapter 5 (Issues facing boys)

Steve Biddulph (2003), *Raising Boys*, 2nd edition, Finch Publishing: Sydney.

Richard Fletcher and Rollo Browne (eds.) (1999), *Boys in Schools*, Finch Publishing: Sydney.

Chapter 6 (Assistance for schools and teachers)

G. DuPaul and J. Stoner (1994), *ADHD in Schools: assessment and intervention strategies*, Guilford Press: New York.

Janet Lerner (1995), *Attention Deficit Disorders: assessment and teaching*, Brooks Cole: Pacific Grove.

Emma Little (2003), *Kids Behaving Badly: teacher strategies for classroom behaviour.* Pearson Education Australia: South Melbourne.

Chapter 7 (The effect of social and cultural forces on ADHD)

Lawrence Diller (1998), *Running on Ritalin*, Bantam Books: New York.

Katherine Ideus, (1994), 'Cultural Foundations of ADHD: a sociological analysis', *Therapeutic Care,* vol.3, no. 2, pp.173–193.

Chapter 8 (ADHD, education policy and health practice)

Ivan Atkinson and Rosalyn Shute (1997). 'Between a rock and a hard place: an Australian perspective on education of children with ADHD,' *Educational and Child Psychology,* 14 (1), pp.21–30.

Brenton Prosser, Robert Reid, Rosalyn Shute and Ivan Atkinson (2002), 'Attention Deficit Hyperactivity Disorder: Special education policy and practice in Australia', *Australian Journal of Education,* 46 (1), pp.65–78.

Ruth Schmidt Neven, Tim Godber and Vicki Anderson (2002), *Rethinking ADHD*, Allen & Unwin: Sydney.

Epilogue

For further reading about my own views and ongoing research, please visit my website: **http://ADHD.bigpondhosting.com/**

Author's notes

A ttention Deficit Hyperactivity Disorder is a complex phenomenon, as is demonstrated by the broad range of academic disciplines that contribute to its conceptualisation and treatment. Within my doctoral dissertation it was necessary to review literature in the fields of: (among others) counselling; cultural studies; education; gender studies; health; literacy; medicine; politics; pharmacology; psychiatry; psychology and sociology. It is beyond the scope of this book to reproduce this review – to do so would detract from the book's core argument. However, I am conscious that because of the diverse and strongly held views about ADHD, it is appropriate to review in detail what various groups believe to be the 'latest' or 'most important' work on ADHD. Accordingly, the following notes provide a starting point for those who wish to explore these elements of ADHD in greater depth.

Page 2: **'Since 1984, the numbers of Australian children using medication for ADHD ...'**: Berbatis, C. G., Sunderland, V. B. and Bulsara, M. 2002, 'Licit psychostimulant consumption in Australia, 1984–2000: international and jurisdictional comparisons', *Medical Journal of Australia,* vol.177, no. 10, pp. 539.

Page 4: **'...it has been estimated that up to 25 percent of males in prison have ADHD ...'**: National Health and Medical Research Council 1997, *Attention Deficit Hyperactivity Disorder*, Australian Government Publishing Service, Canberra, p. 101.

Page 4: **'... our understanding of ADHD has come mostly from medical research'**: The pioneer of medical and psychological understandings of ADHD is Russell Barkley. His influence on the understanding of the cognitive and physiological aspects of ADHD cannot be underestimated. For a more detailed overview of his work, please see the Author's notes for pages 51 and 117.

Page 8: **'As far as medicine is concerned, most researchers now agree ...'**: The medical view is most prominently expressed by Barkley, R. A. 1998, *Attention Deficit Hyperactivity Disorder: a Handbook for Diagnosis and Treatment*, 2nd edn, Guilford Press, New York; while alternative medical views are expressed by Diller, L. 1998, *Running on Ritalin: a physician reflects on children, society and performance in a pill*, Bantam Books, New York.

Page 8: '... a subtle difference in the parts of the brain': An emphasis on subtle differences in the brain is the basis of the neurofeedback approach to ADHD treatment. Neurofeedback makes brainwaves perceptible through the use of sensors attached to the head, which help the brain to improve its ability to regulate bodily function. Brain activity is mapped using an EEG (Electroencephalogram) and patients participate in activities (such as video games) which encourage desired forms of brain activity. Currently, there is not consistent scientific evidence to demonstrate that young people with ADHD have different brains to their non-ADHD peers, or differing brain activity. Until such evidence is found the verdict on neurofeedback will be inconclusive – although the Australian Research Council (ARC) is currently funding industry-linked research into brain profiling. For more information on:

- Neurofeedback: see http://www.eegspectrum.com/IntroToNeuro/.
- ARC research: see http://www.femail.com.au/adhd_a_new_approach.htm

Page 10: 'Journalist Jonathan King (from the *Sydney Morning Herald*) ...':** Taken from an article by Jonathan King on the life of Peter Casserly in the *Sydney Morning Herald* on 11 November 2004 (http://www.smh.com.au/articles/2004/11/10/1100021877985.html).

Page 10: 'Or, as American ADHD expert Dr Lawrence Diller reflects: "I worry about an America where there's no place for an unmedicated Pippi Longstocking or Tom Sawyer." ': Diller, L. 2002. *Should I medicate my child?* Basic Books, New York, p. 222.

Page 11: 'While recent UK research, for instance, has found that children who eat fresh, unprocessed food ...': Taken from an article by Rebecca Smithers in *The Guardian*, 29 November 2004 (http://society.guardian.co.uk/publichealth/story/0,11098,1361889,00.html).

Page 11: '... some children are sensitive to some substances in food': Food additives, food dyes and high levels of sugar can all have an influence on ADHD behaviour. While the consensus among medical research affirms that hyperactivity resulting from dietary factors or food intolerance does not fit the ADHD classification, it is important to note the ongoing work of Susan Dengate in this area. See Dengate, S. (2004), *Fed up with ADHD*, Random House: Sydney; Dengate, S. (1996), *Different Kids: Growing Up with Attention-deficit Disorder*, Random House: Sydney.

Page 13: **'Those who decide against drug use'** and **'those who opt for drug use':** A constant stream of academic papers explores the implications of drug use for ADHD – far too many to review comprehensively in this book. What can be said is that research remains inconclusive on treatment for ADHD: the consensus among ADHD reviews and guidelines is to support a multi-modal treatment approach, but some studies have questioned the utility of a multi-modal approach without medication. There is also ongoing concern among ADHD experts about the lack of research evidence for the efficacy of multi-modal treatment generally: see National Institute of Mental Health Collaborative Multimodal Treatment Study of Children with ADHD (the MTA Cooperative Group) 1999, 'A 14-month randomized clinical trial of treatment strategies for Attention-Deficit/ Hyperactivity Disorder', *Archives of General Psychiatry*, vol.56, pp.1073–1086 (http://archpsyc.ama-assn.org/cgi/content/abstract/56/12/1073).

Conversely, other research has questioned whether drug treatment works or is safe in the longer term. See McDonagh, M.S. & Peterson, K. 2005, *Drug Class Review on Pharmacologic Treatments for ADHD*, final report, September, Oregon Health & Science University: Portland (http://www.abc.net.au/news/ indepth/featureitems/s1464290.htm).

With this in mind, anecdotal evidence and most literature suggests that drug treatment makes a significant and immediate difference to behaviour. The overall result is a situation where drug use as part of a multi-modal response currently remains the preferred treatment model.

Page 24: **"We make no claim to knowing all the answers to the problems of ADHD.":** Reid, R., Maag, J.W. and Vasa, S. F. 1994, 'Attention Deficit Hyperactivity Disorder as a Disability Category: a critique', *Exceptional Children,* vol.60, no. 3, pp. 209.

Page 25: **'US research found that parents have their children tested for ADHD':** See Damico, J. S. and Augustine, L. E. 1995, 'Social Consideration in the Labeling of Students as Attention Deficit Hyperactivity Disordered', *Seminars in Speech and Language,* vol.16, no. 4, pp. 259–274.

Page 25: **'US ADHD specialist Dr Lawrence Diller, author of *Running on Ritalin*, remembers this exchange with a worried mother.':** Diller, L. 1998, *Running on Ritalin*, p. 3.

Page 30: **'The *DSM-IV* checklist':** See American Psychiatric Association 1994, *Diagnostic and Statistical Manual of Mental Disorders, (DSM-IV)*, Fourth Edition; 2000, Fourth Edition Technical Revision (*DSM-IV-TR*), American Psychiatric Association, Washington.

Page 31: '... or other disorders': Research from the University of Tasmania suggests that too many children are being diagnosed with ADHD and suggests that this may mask another motor coordination condition called Developmental Coordination Disorder. See: http://www.abc.net.au/news/newsitems/200510/s1493582.htm.

Page 34: '... dexamphetamine has been used more in Australia': Early anecdotal evidence suggests that the listing of Ritalin in the Australian Pharmaceutical Benefits Scheme in late 2005 is changing this situation; however, it is still too soon for research to verify this trend.

Page 34: 'This is a point reinforced by New Zealand having a significantly higher use of methylphenidate when both drugs are subsidised.': Pharmaceutical Management Agency New Zealand 2003. *Annual Review* (www.pharmac.govt.nz), p. 19.

Page 34: 'In New Zealand, both methylphenidate and dexamphetamine have been eligible for government subsidy ...': Farquhar, S., Fawcett, P. and Fountain, J. 2002, 'Illicit Intravenous Use of Methylphenidate (Ritalin)' *Australian Emergency Nursing Journal*, vol 5, no. 2, p. 25.

Page 34: 'However, the situation changed in Australia in August 2005 when it was announced that methylphenidate would be included in the PBS.': see Health Minister Tony Abbott's Ministerial Press Release 1/8/2005 (http://www.health.gov.au/internet/ministers/publishing.nsf/Content/health-mediarel-yr2005-ta-abb093.htm).

Page 35: 'If only it were that simple – but a crucial study ... in the late 1970s gave psychostimulants to hyperactive boys as well as to boys with no behavioural problems.': See Rappaport, J. and Buschbaum, M. 1980, 'Dextroamphetamine: its cognitive and behavioral effects in normal and hyperactive boys and normal men', *Archives of General Psychiatry,* vol.37, pp.933–943.

Page 36: 'This view, however, is not without its critics, as was demonstrated in recent research from the National Institute of Mental Health in the US.': See National Institute of Mental Health Collaborative Multimodal Treatment Study of Children with ADHD (the MTA Cooperative Group) 1999. 'A 14-month randomised clinical trial of treatment strategies for Attention-Deficit/Hyperactivity Disorder', *Archives of General Psychiatry,* vol.56, pp.1073–1086.

Page 37: 'Internationally, drug use across ten Western countries grew on average by 12 percent between 1994 and 2000.': Berbatis, C. G., Sunderland, V. B. and Bulsara, M., pp.539-540.

Page 37: '... the only two countries to be warned by the United Nations': In early 2006, the US Food and Drug Administration advisory panel issued a further warning in relation to drug treatment. See Pirani, C., *The Australian*, 11/2/06:   http://www.theaustralian.news.com.au/common/story_page/ 0,5744,18109652%255E2702,00.html.

Page 37: The statistics cited in this paragraph are drawn from the following studies: Atkinson, I. M., Robinson, J. A. and Shute, R. 1997, 'Between a rock and a hard place: an Australian perspective on education of children with ADHD', *Educational and Child Psychology*, vol.14, no. 1, pp. 21-30; Manne, A. 2002, 'Children, ADHD and the Contemporary Conditions of Childhood' in *Cries Unheard: a new look at Attention Deficit Hyperactivity Disorder*, eds. Halasz, G.,Anaf, G., Ellingsen, P., Manne,A. and Salo, F.T., Common Press,Altona, pp. 7-28; Morrow, R., Morrow, A., and Haislip, G. 1998, 'Methylphenidate in the United States, 1990 through 1995', *American Journal of Public Health*, vol.88, no.7, p. 1121; Prosser, B. 1999, *Behaviour Management of Management Behaviour? A sociological study of Attention Deficit Hyperactivity Disorder in Australian and American secondary schools*, Bedford Park (SA): Flinders University of South Australia, unpublished doctoral thesis; Prosser, B. and Reid, R. 1999, 'Psychostimulant Use for Children with ADHD in Australia' *Journal of Emotional and Behavioral Disorders*, vol.7, no. 2, pp. 110-117; Reid, R., Hakendorf, P. and Prosser, B. 2002, 'Use of Psychostimulant Medication for ADHD in South Australia', *Journal of the American Academy of Child and Adolescent Psychiatry*, vol.41, no. 8, pp.1-8.

Page 37: 'The growth in Ritalin use in New Zealand started a few years later, but between 1992 and 2003 prescriptions rose from just under 3000 to almost 70,000 ...': Pharmaceutical Management Agency New Zealand 2003. *Annual Review* (www.pharmac.govt.nz), p. 19.

Page 38: 'Growth in PBS prescriptions dispensed for dexamphetamine sulfate': This and the following table taken from Commonwealth Government of Australia, 2004. Issues Brief 8 2004-05: *Medication for AD/HD*, November; Australian Bureau of Statistics, Australian Demographic Statistics, December 2003 (ABS 3101.0).

Page 42: '**In the UK, levels have been estimated as low as one percent, while estimates in the US have been as high as 23 percent.**': See Shaywitz, S. and Shaywitz, B. 1988. 'Attention Deficit Disorder: current perspectives' in J. Kavanagh and T. Truss Jnr. (Eds.), *Learning Disabilities: proceedings of the national conference*. Parkton, New Work Press, pp. 69-523.

Page 42: '**This is true of Australia and New Zealand, where the commonly accepted figure is three to five percent of school-aged children.**' See *DSM-IV*. Australian studies show prevalence rates varying between 2.3-6 percent (National Health and Medical Research Council 1997. *Attention Deficit Hyperactivity Disorder*, Australian Government Publishing Service, Canberra, p.12), with my research in Adelaide showing 2.3 percent (see Prosser, B. and Reid, R. 1999, 'Psychostimulant Use for Children with ADHD in Australia' *Journal of Emotional and Behavioral Disorders*, vol.7, no. 2, pp.110-117), and a recent study in Western Australia showing 4.4 percent (see Berbatis, C. G., Sunderland, V. B. and Bulsara, M. 2002). New Zealand studies show prevalence of 1.4-13.3 percent, although one study in Dunedin showed a prevalence of 6.7 percent (Ministry of Health NZ (2001), *New Zealand Guidelines for the Assessment and Treatment of Attention Deficit/Hyperactivity Disorder*, Wellington: NZ Ministry of Health, p. 6). Notably prevalence in the UK is less than 1 percent (see British Psychological Society 1996, *Attention Deficit Hyperactivity Disorder (ADHD): a psychological response to an evolving concept*, BPS, Leicester).

Page 43: '**... when other causes of similar behaviour are confused:**' For example, Developmental Coordination Disorder (see Author's note for page 31).

Page 45: Quote from US ADHD researcher Dr Katherine Ideus: Ideus, K. 1994, 'Cultural Foundations of ADHD: a sociological analysis', *Therapeutic Care,* vol.3, no. 2, pp. 178.

Page 46: '**... the idea of difficult behaviours being caused by a brain syndrome**' and '**George Still**': The first recorded notion of difficult behaviours originating in a disease or syndrome was made by Heinrich Hoffman in 1854. However, it is the work of George Still that is usually cited as the foundation of the modern conception of ADHD. See Still, G.F. 1902, 'Some abnormal physical conditions in children: the Goulstonian lectures', *Lancet*, vol.1, pp.1008-1012. George Still posited that children who exhibit behaviours we would now call ADHD had a moral deficiency due to a depletion of cell nutrition in the brain. The label used by Still was 'a morbid deficit in moral control'.

Page 48: 'Reflecting on this development almost 20 years later, a leading US researcher in this area, Dr Maurice Laufer, claimed ...': Quoted in Schachar, R. 1986, 'Hyperkinetic Syndrome: historical development of the concept' in *The Overactive Child*, ed. E. Taylor, Blackwell, Oxford, pp. 27.

Page 50: ' ... made the term Attention Deficit Disorder (ADD) official': Not all those within the psychiatric discipline accept the condition ADHD. One notable exception is those working within the psychodynamic approach, who argue that while a range of children's behavioural characteristics may be viewed as 'symptoms' – thereby earning the child the diagnostic label of ADHD – such symptoms are not sufficient by themselves to diagnose children as ill, much less to justify medicating them. They claim that a failure to make a 'holistic' assessment of a child within a family context, as well as within his or her wider school and social settings, may result in a misdiagnosis of behaviour as illness. See Halasz, G., Anaf, G., Ellingsen, P., Manne, A. and Salo, F. T. (Eds.) (2002), *Cries Unheard: a new look at Attention Deficit Hyperactivity Disorder*, Common Press, Altona.

Pages 50-51: '... released his book *Attention Deficit Hyperactivity Disorder*': Russell Barkley's approach to ADHD is encapsulated in the following extract:

> 'ADHD must be viewed as a developmentally disabling disorder of inattention, behavioural disinhibition, and the regulation of activity level to situational demands. The evidence accumulating in the past ten years has more than proven this initial view to be correct; indeed, it is the only humane perspective on this disorder.' (Barkley, R.A. 1990, *Attention Deficit Hyperactivity Disorder: A handbook for diagnosis and treatment*, Guilford Press: New York, p.ix).

In his book, Barkley argued that ADHD is a genetically-inherited physiological condition that first limits a child's inhibition and then progresses into developmental disorders of social control and attention. He also made the argument for a distinction between inattention and hyperactivity. During the late Nineties, Barkley re-conceptualised ADHD as primarily a lack of ability and motivation to follow rules, referring to it also as 'Developmental Delay in Self-Control' (this label has yet to gain wider acceptance). The clarity of Barkley's explanations about the cause of the disorder and how medication impacted on cognitive function was a catalyst to the significant growth in professional and popular awareness of the disorder in the US. His book also became part of a significant change in Australia where, throughout the Eighties, ADHD had not been widely recognised or diagnosed and treated with psychostimulant medication. Barkley's handbook on ADHD became well known and was cited as an authority on the disorder, its genetic transmission, its cognitive implications and the appropriateness of psychostimulant treatment. The book also inspired several popular texts for parents that appeared in Australian bookstores in the early Nineties. However, it would be misleading to attribute the change in Australian awareness of the ADHD label solely to the appearance of these books; it is also important to locate the changes within other changes in the Australian political and cultural landscape at the time (see Chapters 7 & 8).

For my part, Barkley's work made me more sensitive to the physiological aspects of ADHD; much of my own work on the social aspects of ADHD has developed in parallel with his arguments about its physical and cognitive aspects. Recently, Barkley gave greater recognition to this social side of ADHD, but he still maintains a focus on the individual, the parent and the school. In this book, I consider the broader social, cultural, political and structural influences at work. As such, I see myself contributing to the other side of the ADHD coin.

While this summary provides an introduction to the core ideas contributed by Russell Barkley, it does not purport to be a comprehensive or an up-to-date overview. A good starting point for those wanting to explore his work for the first time is: Barkley, R. A. (2005), *Taking Charge of ADHD: The Complete, Authoritative Guide for Parents,* 3rd Edition, Guilford Press: New York. Another text that is useful for developing a deeper understanding of his work (including his recent research) is: Barkley, R. A. (2006), *Attention Deficit Hyperactivity Disorder: A handbook for diagnosis and treatment,* 3rd Edition, Guilford Press: New York.

Page 53: **'As some disability researchers point out …':** Influential in the area of 'Disability Theory' is the work of Oliver. See Oliver, M. 1990, *The Politics of Disablement: A sociological approach.* St. Martin's Press: New York. At the core of Oliver's argument was the idea that if disability was understood as an individual tragedy, then policy and treatment would reflect this to focus on healing the individual. In contrast, if disability was understood socially, then policy and treatment would need to address problems in the social structure. Oliver also argued that there was an underlying logic to the development of capitalism which actually created a medical and individual problem labelled 'disabled' as a response to changing work organisation, social relations and family demands. He further criticised medical approaches for constructing a 'disability' label that was partial and failed to take into account wider issues; and for setting up a system of policies and services that reinforce medical labels and their negative social ramifications. Although ADHD is not a disability, such insights have clear implications for the discourses surrounding ADHD and how they shape conceptions of what the condition is and how it is best treated.

Also significant in this field is the work of Bart. See Bart, D.S. 1984, 'The Differential Diagnosis of Special Education: managing social pathology as individual disability', L. Barton & S. Tomlinson (Eds.), *Special Education as Social Interests* (pp. 81–121), Croom Helm: London. Bart attempted to consider issues such as labelling, disability and integration, particularly in relation to schools. She argued that special education rarely acted to break down barriers, but only accommodated the disabled within existing (limited) notions of normality. She claimed that the language of special education was overtly ideological and the very use of terms such as 'disability' and 'inclusion' were barriers to integration. Bart also noted a pattern in the development of specialist areas, which become legitimised and then reinforced by the same medical specialists. Thus, she identified a need to survive within the medical paradigm which relies on ongoing diagnosis and labelling.

page 53: **'Labeling Theory':** For an introduction to 'Labeling Theory', see: Becker, H. S. 1964, *The Other Side*, Free Press: New York; Becker, H. S. (1973), 'Labeling Theory Reconsidered', H. S. Becker (Ed.), *Outsiders: Studies in the Sociology of Deviance,* (pp. 177–208), Free Press: New York; Rist, R. C. (1977), 'On Understanding the Processes of Schooling: the contribution of labeling theory', J. Karabel & A. H. Halsley (Eds.), *Power and Ideology in Education,* Oxford Uni Press: New York, pp. 292–305.

Page 54: **Social researcher Peter Conrad used "Labeling Theory"**: Conrad, P. 1976, *Identifying Hyperactive Children: the medicalization of deviant behavior*, D.C. Heath & Co., US, p. 89.

Page 54: **'From the history of ADHD presented above, it is tempting to do what ADHD critic Thomas Armstrong does':** Armstrong, T. 1997, *The Myth of the ADD Child,* Plume Books, New York, p. 10.

Page 55: **'More recently, there has been a growth in the use of antidepressant drugs for psychological and social problems ...':** Diller, L. 1998, *Running on Ritalin*, p. 108.

Page 56: **'... in 1995 Ciba-Geigy...':** Diller, L. 1998, *Running on Ritalin,* p. 39.

Page 57: **' "Can we make a video about ADHD and send it to "A Current Affair" and show Ray Martin that he's crap?" ':** It would be a mistake to read these student views as an attack on either Ray Martin or the Nine program 'A Current Affair'. This program and its host were known to the students because they are icons in the Australian current affairs genre. Rather, these comments are a challenge to all current affairs media to forgo sensationalism and talk to young people like Charlie about 'what it's actually like' to live with ADHD.

Page 59: **'Another crucial development in the media history of ADHD was a 1994 *Time* magazine article':** Wallis, C. 1994. 'Life in Overdrive', *Time*, 18 July.

Page 59: **'... a trend highlighted by a 1998 story – again in *Time*... ':** Gibbs, N. 1998. 'The Age of Ritalin', *Time*, 30 November.

Page 61: **'There is little doubt about the effect the media has had on ADHD in the United States':** This quote is from Diller, L. 1998, *Running on Ritalin*, p. 35.

Page 61: **'... contribute to the growth of a popular understanding of the disorder':** In addition to the information provided by television and the Internet in the US, there is currently a strong emphasis on ADHD in women's and health insurance magazines in that nation. Some would argue that this popular awareness has led to a risk of ADHD overdiagnosis (see pages 42-44).

Page 64: **'Previous studies have shown how information about ADHD spread across Western countries':** For more information see Safer, D. J., & Krager, J. M. 1984, 'Trends in Medication Therapy for Hyperactivity: national and international perspectives', *Advances in Learning and Behavioral Disabilities*, 3, pp. 125-149.

Page 75: **'You got a "U".':** 'U' stands for 'unsatisfactory' or 'unfinished; it is the lowest grade that can be given to an assignment.

Page 83: **'I got a week of binnies and an after-school for that.':** 'binnies' is a student colloquialism for picking up litter and putting it in the bin for detention.

Page 88: **'He had a lot of micro machines':** 'Micro machines' are small mechanical toys that convert from robots into vehicles, not unlike the well-known product 'Transformers'.

Page 93: **'Needs beyond literacy and numeracy':** This point does not seek to draw attention away from the importance of literacy and numeracy support for young people with ADHD. Rather, it seeks to reinforce the importance of behavioural and social skill barriers that might form an obstacle to such support or remedial strategies. The importance of literacy is demonstrated by work with adolescents that shows support to improve reading can help reduce behaviour management problems. For instance, the experience of Professor Vicki Anderson at Melbourne's Royal Children's Hospital points to the inattention of many students being a secondary problem to their failure to learn how to read. See Milburn, C., 'Children in crisis: the real diagnosis', *The Age*, 6/12/04. (http://www.theage.com.au/news/National/Children in-crisis-the-real-diagnosis/2004/12/05/1102182155642.html).

This point is further emphasised by research findings linking early success in literacy with improved self-esteem and greater attentive behaviour. See Rowe, K.J. & Rowe, K.S. 1999, 'Chapter 5: implications of the findings' *International Journal of Educational Research*, 31, pp.65–80. This research also suggests that growth in the use of 'in context' and 'authentic' pedagogies requires greater sustained attention from students, which may have inadvertently lifted the premium on attentive behaviour in schooling. In response, it argues for more use of structured early literacy interventions by teachers to reduce the need for behavioural modifications. Such recommendations should be considered in the context of contemporary public and academic debates about 'traditional' versus 'progressive' emphases within literacy teaching in Australia, as well as research that highlights that the general implementation of 'connected' pedagogies remains patchy. See Luke, A. et al. 2003, *Beyond the Middle: a report about literacy and numeracy development of target group students in the middle years of schooling*, Griffith University: Brisbane. With this in mind, it is evident that more early intervention with targeted pedagogical strategies to improve learning and a learners' self-esteem are needed, and can only enhance a 'skills not pills' response to ADHD.

Page 99: 'As Natasha Stott Despoja, the former Australian Democrats' leader, explains': See Stott-Despoja, N. 1997, *Speech to the Australian Constitutional Convention*, Parliament House, Canberra, 18 June.

Page 102: 'In Australia, boys are four to nine times more likely than girls ...': National Health and Medical Research Council 1997. *Attention Deficit Hyperactivity* Disorder, Australian Government Publishing Service, Canberra, p. 14; and Manne, A. 2002, 'Children, ADHD and the Contemporary Conditions of Childhood' in *Cries Unheard: a new look at Attention Deficit Hyperactivity Disorder*, p. 9.

Page 103: 'US research has shown that boys are not only more likely to be diagnosed with ADHD ...': See Reid, R. and Katsiyannis, A. 1995, 'Attention

Deficit/Hyperactivity Disorder and Section 504', *Remedial and Special Education,* vol.16, no. 1, pp.44–52.

Page 103: **'Similar research in Australia has shown that many young people with social skill needs fall through the policy support cracks.':** See Atkinson, I. M., Robinson, J.A. and Shute, R. 1997.

Page 109: **'Research shows that if we keep boys at school longer, the quality and quantity of work they later have improves.':** See Lingard, B., Martino, W., Mills, M., and Bahr, M. 2003, *Addressing the educational needs of boys.* Commonwealth of Australia: Commonwealth Department of Education, Science and Training; and see also Lingard, B., Mills, M., Hayes, D. 2000. 'Teachers School Reform and Social Justice: challenging research and practice'. *Australian Educational Researcher,* vol.27, no.3, pp. 99–115.

Page 110: **'While figures once suggested that about five boys for every one girl were diagnosed ...':** See Reid, R., Hakendorf, P. and Prosser, B. 2002, 'Use of Psychostimulant Medication for ADHD in South Australia', *Journal of the American Academy of Child and Adolescent Psychiatry,* vol.41, no. 8, pp. 1–8.

Page 110: **'...some experts suggest that it could be partly explained by the way ADHD is studied and diagnosed.':** A number of researchers have commented on this issue: Barkley, R.A. 1995, 'A closer look at the *DSM-IV* criteria for ADHD: some unresolved issues', *ADHD report,* vol. 3, no. 3, pp. 1–5; Bussing, R., Schoenberg, N.E., Rogers, K.M., Zima, B.T. and Angus, S. 1998b, 'Explanatory Models of ADHD: do they differ by ethnicity, child gender, or treatment status?', *Journal of Emotional and Behavioral Disorders,* vol. 6, pp. 233–242; and Reid, R., Hakendorf, P. and Prosser, B. 2002.

Page 111: **'As Dr Lawrence Diller puts it, "boys tend to act out, while girls tend to act in" ':** Diller, L. 2002. *Should I medicate my child?,* p. 175.

Page 111: **'If a society puts half its children in dresses and skirts but warns them not to move in ways that reveal their underpants ...':** See Vines, G. 1993, *Raging Hormones: Do They Rule Our Lives?* Virago, London.

Page 113: **'In general, studies show that boys don't perform as well as girls, and find English less interesting.':** See Alloway, N., Freebody, P. Gilbert, P. and Muspratt, S. 2002, *Boys, literacy and schooling: Expanding the repertoires of practice.* Commonwealth of Australia: Curriculum Corporation and Commonwealth Department of Education, Science and Training.

Page 117: '**... and learning strategies to make the space for big-picture progress**': Notably, Russell Barkley has highlighted that many students with ADHD do not demonstrate poorer academic achievement and learning difficulty; however, it is still important to consider a range of resources that can inform teachers' pedagogy in relation to those students with ADHD who do struggle at school. I wish to briefly mention four of these:

1) One pedagogical resource is Barkley's work on the cognitive implications for ADHD and learning. See: Barkley, R. A. 1998, *Attention Deficit Hyperactivity Disorder:A handbook for diagnosis and treatment*, 2nd Edition, Guilford Press: New York; Barkley, R. 1997, 'Behavioral inhibition, sustained attention, and executive functions: Constructing a unifying theory of ADHD', *Psychological Bulletin, 121*, pp.65–94; Barkley, R. 1996, 'The North American perspective on Attention Deficit Hyperactivity Disorder', *The Australian Educational and Developmental Psychologist, 13*(1), pp.2–23.These insights have been influential among educational psychologists in Australia and North America, including Kathy Baker. Her research has found that the problems with core cognitive functions identified by Barkley can result in reading disabilities. From this research she has developed a reading intervention method for students, the pedagogies of which could be used by teachers to develop strategies for supporting other academic areas, behaviour and social skills. See: Baker, K. 2004, *Reading Success: A reading intervention for students with ADHD,* Hawker Brownlow Education: Moorabin, Vic; Baker, K. 2001, 'Attention Deficit Hyperactivity Disorder and reading achievement', *Queensland Journal of Educational Research*, 17, 1, pp. 68–84.

2) Another model that offers teachers a range of pedagogical resources is the 'functional' or 'goodness of fit' approach (which has been more prominent among educational psychologists in the UK). From this perspective, behaviour is viewed not as the result of some disorder inherent to the individual, but is conceptualised as resulting from the combination of an individual's skills (or lack thereof) and environmental factors. From this perspective, an ADHD label (or any other, for that matter) is irrelevant. The sole focus of functional assessment is identifying the causal basis or functional relationship between problem behaviour, the environment and the individual's repertoire of skills (see hint 18 on page 119). One of the greatest benefits of the functional approach is that research has demonstrated that teachers can perform functional assessment and practically implement it in the classroom.The following texts are useful for further information on functional approaches to ADHD: Maag, J., & Reid, R. 1994, 'Attention Deficit-Hyperactivity Disorder: a functional approach to assessment and treatment', *Behavioral Disorders*, 20, pp.5–23; Reid, R. 1996, 'Three Faces

of Attention-Deficit Hyperactivity Disorder'. *Journal of Child and Family Studies*, 5, pp.249–265; Reid, R., Reason, R., Maag, J., Prosser, B., & Xu, C. 1998. 'Attention Deficit Hyperactivity Disorder: a perspective on perspectives', *Educational and Child Psychology*, 15, pp.56–67.

3) A lesser-known pedagogical resource is the use of narrative therapy methods when working with students with ADHD. Often a focus on behaviour management in schools can reframe students with problems in schooling as 'problem students', with ADHD being one prominent example of such a deficit identity. Using the idea that a person's identity is a narrative, Nylund and Corsiglia defined ADHD as a self-narrative that emphasises individual deficit and failure. In response, they sought to wrest back ownership of the label for the individual by rewriting it as a positive self-narrative. They proposed that a young person should be encouraged to reclaim their gifts and talents, not lose them to a label. See Nylund, D., & Corsiglia, V. 1997, 'From Deficits to Special Abilities: working narratively with children labeled ADHD' in M. Hoyt (Ed.), *Constructive Therapies 2* (pp. 163–183), Guilford: New York. Similarly, Ian Law describes his use of narrative therapy with young people diagnosed with ADHD to deconstruct the dominant conception of ADHD, thus allowing more scope for the discovery of strengths and success. See Law, I. 1997, 'Therapy with a Shoddily Built Construct', in D. Nylund & C. Smith (Eds.), *Narrative Therapies with Children and Teens* (pp. 282–306), Guilford Press: New York. An explanation of the pedagogical possibilities for narrative therapy can be found in the work considering 'students at risk' by Fitzclarence and Hickey, see: Hickey, C. & Fitzclarence, L. 2004, 'Regimes of risk: the need for a pedagogy for peer groups', *Asia-Pacific Journal of Teacher Education*, 32 (1), pp.49–63; Fitzclarence, L. & Hickey, C. 1999, 'The construction of a responsible self-identity: the why and what of narrative pedagogy', Australian Association for Research in Education Annual Conference, Melbourne. Their consideration of pedagogy is best understood as the learning that results from the processes of narration and re-narration of identity, rather than the implementation of specific pedagogical strategies.

4) Finally, the book by DuPaul and Stoner (see Appendix B) provides a comprehensive orientation to pedagogies that can be used with ADHD by teachers.

Page 117: **'100 helpful hints for teachers':** The following 'helpful hints' are drawn from my experience working with young people diagnosed with ADHD as a youth worker, teacher and researcher, as well as many discussions on the issue with teaching colleagues. The foundation of these practical suggestions is anecdotal and experiential; they are not presented as the result of rigorous empirical research either by me or others working in the area of pedagogical research. However, these 'hints' are offered as a resource for teachers of students with ADHD and may be useful in different teaching contexts, at different times or with different students.

Page 122: **'Consider providing students with a keyring USB ...':** This is a small storage device that can plug into the USB port of any computer, and is now available in the form of a keyring with substantial memory and at a reasonable price.

Page 125: **'According to Western Australian research, 35–50 percent of children with ADHD have to repeat a year ...':** See Carragher, G.L. 2003. *Life after diagnosis: The social experience of adolescents diagnosed with attention-deficit/hyperactivity disorder and how they manage their lives*, Mount Lawley (WA): Edith Cowan University Education Faculty, unpublished doctoral thesis.

Page 126: **'The first such influence is what Australian education expert, Professor John Smyth, calls the "welding of education onto the economy."** ': This notion is discussed in a number of texts including Smyth, J., Hattam, R. and Lawson, M. (Eds.) 1998, *Schooling for a Fair Go*, The Federation Press, Sydney; Smyth, J. 2001, *Critical Politics of Teachers' Work*, Peter Lang, New York; and Thomson, P. 2002, *Schooling the Rustbelt Kids: making the difference in changing times*, Allen & Unwin, Sydney.

Page 127: **'University of Nottingham Professor (and ex-South Australian school principal) Pat Thomson talks about the "virtual schoolbag" that every child brings with them.':** See Thomson, p. 2002.

Page 132: **'Professor Roger Slee ... argues that as government policies call for higher retention rates in schools ...':** See Slee, R. 1994, 'Finding a Student Voice in School Reform: student disaffection, pathologies of disruption and educational control', *International Studies in the Sociology of Education*, vol. 4, no. 2, pp. 147–172.

Page 132: **' "As the contexts of young people and the expectations for their schooling become more complex ..." ':** Slee, pp. 147–8.

Page 133: **'When one considers American research that shows that parents only seek out an ADHD diagnosis after giving up on getting support from schools ...':** That parents seek out an ADHD diagnosis after giving up on school support was demonstrated by Damico, J. S. and Augustine, L. E. 1995; while the notion of blaming the individual for the problem can be found in the work of Professor Roger Slee (see Bibliography).

Page 135: Chapter 7, 'ADHD and society': This chapter provides an introduction to some of the insights that sociology can offer our understanding of ADHD. As this book is written for young people, parents, teachers and the community, a scholarly and comprehensive sociological analysis is beyond its scope. However, the following texts (along with those linked to this chapter in Appendix B) offer further sociological consideration of ADHD, see: Prosser, B. 2006, *Seeing Red: a case of critical narrative in ADHD research*, PostPressed: Flaxton; Prosser, B. 1999, 'Behaviour Management of Management Behaviour? A sociological study of Attention Deficit Hyperactivity Disorder in Australian and American secondary schools', doctoral dissertation, Bedford Park: Flinders University of South Australia.

Page 135: **"In the reality of the workaday world, the individual is expected to cope with society ..."**: Smelter, R., Rasch, B., Fleming, J., Nazos, P. and Baranowski, S. 1996. 'Is Attention Deficit Disorder Becoming A Desired Diagnosis?', *Phi Delta Kappan*, vol. 77, no. 16, p. 432.

Page 136: **'... little attention has been given to why ADHD has exploded in some parts of some societies'**: It is important to note here the Australian work of Halasz et. al., who have considered how changing social and economic parameters have led to an increase in the diagnosis of ADHD in children. See Halasz, G., Anaf, G., Ellingsen, P., Manne, A. and Salo, F. T. (Eds.) (2002), *Cries Unheard: a new look at Attention Deficit Hyperactivity Disorder*, Common Press, Altona.

Page 136, Page 144: ADHD and Asia: One explanation of the lack of prevalence of ADHD among Asian communities in Australia is that the philosophy that underpins ADHD is predominantly Western. As a result, current ADHD theory does not provide the conceptual links necessary to be applied to traditional Asian cultures. However, as new generations of Asian communities contribute to multicultural Australia, and countries such as China increasingly embrace the West, this area provides a fascinating opportunity for future ADHD research.

Page 137: **'Although there is a lack of data on prevalence among Maori children ...'**: Ministry of Health NZ (2001), *New Zealand Guidelines for the Assessment and Treatment of Attention Deficit/Hyperactivity Disorder*, Wellington: NZ Ministry of Health, p. 6.

Page 137: 'Yet there's also new evidence that while Afro-American children are less likely to get a diagnosis and treatment ...': See Bussing, R., Schoenberg, N.E., Rogers, K.M., Zima, B.T. and Angus, S. 1998b; and also Maurer, K. 1996, 'African-American Children Less Likely to Get Ritalin', *Clinical Psychiatry News*, vol.24, pp. 1-2.

Page 138: 'It could be that as Australia mirrored a shift towards conservatism in American politics ...': See Ideus, K. 1994, 'Cultural Foundations of ADHD: a sociological analysis', *Therapeutic Care*, vol.3, no. 2, pp. 173-193.

Page 139: "The pragmatic, reductionist stance which has come to dominate the ADHD field in the United States ...": Ideus, K. 1994, pp. 179.

Page 139: 'However, in my research in Australia there appear to be clusters of children using medication ...': See Prosser, B. 1999; and Reid, R., Hakendorf, P. and Prosser, B. 2002.

Page 141: 'In one US study, researcher Gwendolyn Stevens ...': See Stevens, G. 1981, 'Bias in the attribution of hyperkinetic behavior as a function of ethnic identification and socioeconomic status', *Psychology in the Schools*, vol. 18, no. 1, pp. 99-106.

Page 144: '...in the mid-1990s the British Psychological Society estimated that ADHD affected less that one percent of children in the UK...': See British Psychological Society 1996, *Attention Deficit Hyperactivity Disorder (ADHD): a psychological response to an evolving concept*, BPS, Leicester.

Page 144: 'In Europe, diagnosis and drug use for ADHD is significantly lower in the UK, Spain and Holland ...': See Berbatis, C. G., Sunderland, V. B. and Bulsara, M. 2002, pp. 539-543.

Page 144: '... as Professor Paul Cooper of Cambridge University points out, levels are lower in the UK ...': See Cooper, P. and Ideus, K. 1995, 'Attention Deficit Hyperactivity Disorder: a trojan horse?', *Support for Learning*, vol. 10, no. 1, pp. 29-34.

Page 146: 'Some experts believe ADHD is the result of a mismatch between what a person is capable of and what contemporary society expects of them ...': The functionalist model is discussed in Reid, R., Reason, R., Maag, J., Prosser, B. and Xu, C. 1998, 'Attention Deficit Hyperactivity Disorder: a perspective on perspectives', *Educational and Child Psychology*, vol.15, no.

4, pp.56–67; while Atkinson, I. M., Robinson, J. A. and Shute, R. 1997 elaborates on a similar 'goodness of fit' model.

Page 146: **'Others even suggest that what's different about children with ADHD is that they haven't lost some of the traits that were so useful to our hunter-gatherer ancestors.':** See, for example, Polis, B. 2001, *Only a Mother Could Love Him, ADD:Attention Deficit Disorder,* Seaview Press, Henley Beach.

Page 146: **'... some sociologists suggest that treating ADHD this way can be seen as a kind of social control':** Examples of such sociological views include Conrad, P. 1976; Diller, L. 1998, *Running on Ritalin;* Ideus, K. 1994; and Prosser, B., 2005 (see Bibliography).

Page 147: **'According to the Australia Institute, Australians now work longer hours than the Germans, the Americans, and even the Japanese ...':** Australia Institute, 2004.'Take the rest of the year off', 20 November. (http://www.tai.org.au/WhatsNew_Files/WhatsNew/Overwork%20day%2020th%20November.pdf).

Page 150: **'This thinking shows up in this quote from recent research by Dr. Georgia Carragher on Western Australian adolescents with ADHD':** Carragher, G.L. 2003.

Page 154: Professor Fiona Stanley quote from interview with Andrew Denton on 'Enough Rope', Australian Broadcasting Commission, 6 October 2003.

Page 155: **'If we want to improve our children's mental health, and grow healthy future generations of Australians, she says, governments must put children first ...':** Stanley, F., as above.

Page 155: **'It is a warning echoed by the National Health and Medical Research Council Report into ADHD ...':** See National Health and Medical Research Council 1997.

Page 156: **"ADHD is having a wide impact in Australia.":** Quote from Atkinson, I. M., Robinson, J.A. and Shute, R., p. 22.

Page 160: **'A good example of how this works can be seen in a comment made by Labor Party Senator for WA, Mark Bishop, in 2003':** Bishop, M.

2003,'Motion to the Social Welfare: Carer Allowance', *Senate Hansard*, Canberra, 13 August.

Page 162: **"Students who are depressed, suffering eating disorders, involved in substance abuse …"**: Quote from Thomson, P., 2002.

Page 170: **'The United Nations has warned Australia about our high use of drugs to treat behaviour problems'**: Reported by Moor, K. 1999, 'Drug Fear on hyper kids'. *Herald Sun*, 25 February.

Page 172 (and page 165): **'… the gap between policy and practice in providing services for ADHD'**: One of the arguments made in this book is that American research (which shows that parents seek out an ADHD diagnosis due to frustration at a lack of services and support from schools) aligns with the Australian situation. See Damico, J. S. and Augustine, L. E. 1995, 'Social Consideration in the Labeling of Students as Attention Deficit Hyperactivity Disordered', *Seminars in Speech and Language*, vol.16, no. 4, pp. 259-274. Further, the book notes that the Australian policy situation results in many young people (once diagnosed with ADHD) still falling through the cracks between policy and practice. See: Atkinson, I. M., Robinson, J. A. and Shute, R. 1997, 'Between a rock and a hard place: an Australian perspective on education of children with ADHD', *Educational and Child Psychology*, vol.14, no. 1, pp. 21-30; Prosser, B., Reid, R., Shute, R. & Atkinson, I. 2002, 'Attention Deficit Hyperactivity Disorder: Special education policy and practice in Australia', *Australian Journal of Education*, vol.46, no. 1, pp.65-78.

Aware that there is often a significant time-lag between changes in policy, service provision and the publication of research results that would show their impact, in early 2005 I wrote to representatives of state, Catholic and independent (AIS) education bodies in each Australian state. In my correspondence, I invited each body to present the latest information on the policy and support applicable to students in their schools. The outcome of this review was that, at time of publication, there was neither specific policy nor specific service provision for ADHD, and a situation continues where young people have to qualify for support through other associated learning difficulties or co-morbid disorders.

Page 173: **'Given the Federal Government's interest in boys and schooling – in 2003 it held an inquiry into the needs of boys in school'**: See Lingard, B., Martino, W., Mills, M., and Bahr, M. 2003.

Page 173: '**Professor Bob Lingard from the University of Sheffield, one of the authors of that Commonwealth inquiry, offers an interesting insight into the current economic pressure in education.**': Lingard, B., Mills, M., Hayes, D. 2000.

Appendix A: Source: World Health Organisation [WHO] 1993, *International Classification of Diseases (ICD-10)*, World Health Organisation, Geneva.

Acknowledgements

First and foremost, I would like to thank Paula Goodyear for her sincere encouragement, editorial suggestions and insightful contributions to this book. Without her support, this book may never have come into existence and certainly not in such an accessible form. Thanks also go to Finch Publishing who, after a five-year journey of writing, showed the courage to make this book a reality.

I wish to thank my doctoral supervisor, John Smyth, who gave me the opportunity to devote several years to studying ADHD, as well as the tools to analyse what I discovered. Further, it was his challenge to write a critical sociological text for the shelves of popular bookstores that was behind the genesis of this book. My thanks also go to Pat Thomson from Nottingham University, whose enthusiasm and advice was instrumental in my persisting with the early stages of writing this book.

A special mention must go to Robert Reid at the University of Nebraska, who wisely introduced me to the trials of writing at the same time as the joys of Scotch whisky. His extensive knowledge of ADHD was not only invaluable in forging my broader understanding of the disorder, but also in reviewing the content of this book.

I would also like to acknowledge the Queen's Trust for Young Australians, the Young Australian of the Year Awards, the Flinders University Amy Forwood Award and the University of South Australia – without the generous support of these groups, this book would not have been possible.

Thanks also goes to my wife, Cherie, whose amazing confidence and patient companionship helped me through what was an exhilarating, depressing and at times volatile journey to better understand ADHD.

Finally, my sincere thanks go to the adolescents and their families who bravely shared their stories about living with ADHD and enthusiastically contributed to my research. Without them, this book would not exist, and it is their desire to help those who will follow that makes this book so important.

Bibliography

Alloway, N., Freebody, P. Gilbert, P. and Muspratt, S. 2002, *Boys, literacy and schooling: Expanding the repertoires of practice*. Commonwealth of Australia: Curriculum Corporation and Commonwealth Department of Education, Science and Training.

American Psychiatric Association 1994, *Diagnostic and Statistical Manual of Mental Disorders*, (*DSM-IV*), Fourth Edition; 2000, Fourth Edition Technical Revision (*DSM-IV-TR*), American Psychiatric Association, Washington.

Armstrong, T. 1997, *The Myth of the ADD Child*, Plume Books, New York.

Atkinson, I. M., Robinson, J. A. and Shute, R. 1997, 'Between a rock and a hard place: an Australian perspective on education of children with ADHD', *Educational and Child Psychology*, vol.14, no. 1, pp.21–30.

Barkley, R.A. 1995, 'A closer look at the *DSM-IV* criteria for ADHD: some unresolved issues', *ADHD report*, vol. 3, no. 3, pp. 1–5

Barkley, R. A. 1998, *Attention Deficit Hyperactivity Disorder: a Handbook for Diagnosis and Treatment*, 2nd edn, Guilford Press, New York.

Berbatis, C. G., Sunderland, V. B. and Bulsara, M. 2002, 'Licit psychostimulant consumption in Australia, 1984–2000: international and jurisdictional comparisons', *Medical Journal of Australia*, vol.177, no. 10, pp.539–543.

Biddulph, S. 1997, *Raising Boys*, Finch Publishing, Sydney.

British Psychological Society 1996, *Attention Deficit Hyperactivity Disorder (ADHD): a psychological response to an evolving concept*, BPS, Leicester.

Bussing, R., Zima, B.T., Perwein, A.R., Belin, T.R. and Widawski, M. 1998, 'Attention Deficit Hyperactivity Disorder, use of services and unmet need'. *American Journal of Public Health*, vol.88, pp.880–886.

Bussing, R., Schoenberg, N.E., Rogers, K.M., Zima, B.T. and Angus, S. 1998b, 'Explanatory Models of ADHD: do they differ by ethnicity, child gender, or treatment status?', *Journal of Emotional and Behavioral Disorders*, vol.6, pp.233–242.

Carragher, G.L. 2003. *Life after diagnosis: The social experience of adolescents diagnosed with attention-deficit/hyperactivity disorder and how they manage their lives*,: Edith Cowan University Education Faculty, Mount Lawley (WA), unpublished doctoral thesis.

Commonwealth Government of Australia, 2004. *Issues Brief 8 2004-05: Medication for AD/HD*, November; Australian Bureau of Statistics, *Australian Demographic Statistics*, December 2003 (ABS 3101.0).

Conrad, P. 1976, *Identifying Hyperactive Children: the medicalization of deviant behavior*, D.C. Heath & Co., USA.

Cooper, P. and Ideus, K. 1995, 'Attention Deficit Hyperactivity Disorder: a trojan horse?', *Support for Learning*, vol.10, no. 1, pp.29-34.

Damico, J. S. and Augustine, L. E. 1995, 'Social Consideration in the Labeling of Students as Attention Deficit Hyperactivity Disordered', *Seminars in Speech and Language*, vol.16, no. 4, pp.259-274.

Diller, L. 1998, *Running on Ritalin: a physician reflects on children, society and performance in a pill*, Bantam Books, New York.

Diller, L. 2002. *Should I Medicate my Child?* Basic Books, New York.

Farquhar, S., Fawcett, P. and Fountain, J. 2002, 'Illicit Intravenous Use of Methylphenidate (Ritalin)' *Australian Emergency Nursing Journal*, vol 5, no. 2, p.25.

Gibbs, N. 1998. 'The Age of Ritalin'. *Time Magazine USA*, November 30.

Halasz, G., Anaf, G., Ellingsen, P., Manne, A. and Salo, F.T. eds. 2002, *Cries Unheard: a new look at Attention Deficit Hyperactivity Disorder*, Common Press, Altona.

Hazell, P. L., McDowell, M. J. and Walton, J.M. 1996, 'Management of children prescribed psychostimulant medication for attention deficit hyperactivity disorder in the Hunter region of NSW', *Medical Journal of Australia*, vol.165, pp.477-480.

Ideus, K. 1994, 'Cultural Foundations of ADHD: a sociological analysis', *Therapeutic Care*, vol.3, no. 2, pp.173-193.

Laurence, J., and McCallum, D. 1998, 'The Myth or Reality of Attention Deficit Disorder', *Discourse*, vol.19, no.2, pp.183-200.

Lingard, B., Martino, W., Mills, M., and Bahr, M. 2003, *Addressing the Educational Needs of Boys*. Commonwealth Department of Education, Science and Training: Commonwealth of Australia.

Lingard, B., Mills, M., Hayes, D. 2000. 'Teachers, School Reform and Social Justice: challenging research and practice'. *Australian Educational Researcher*, vol.27, no.3, pp.99-115.

Manne, A. 2002, 'Children, ADHD and the Contemporary Conditions of Childhood' in *Cries Unheard: a new look at Attention Deficit Hyperactivity Disorder*, eds. Halasz, G., Anaf, G., Ellingsen, P., Manne, A. and Salo, F. T., Common Press, Altona, pp.7-28.

Maurer, K. 1996, 'African-American Children Less Likely to Get Ritalin', *Clinical Psychiatry News*, vol.24, pp.1-2.

Ministry of Health NZ (2001), *New Zealand Guidelines for the Assessment and Treatment of Attention Deficit/Hyperactivity Disorder*, NZ Ministry of Health. Wellington.

Morrow, R., Morrow, A., and Haislip, G. 1998, 'Methylphenidate in the United States, 1990 through 1995', *American Journal of Public Health*, vol.88, no.7, p.1121.

National Health and Medical Research Council 1997. *Attention Deficit Hyperactivity Disorder*, Australian Government Publishing Service, Canberra.

National Institute of Mental Health Collaborative Multimodal Treatment Study of Children with ADHD (the MTA Cooperative Group) 1999. 'A 14 month randomized clinical trial of treatment strategies for Attention-Deficit/Hyperactivity Disorder', *Archives of General Psychiatry*, vol.56, pp.1073–1086.

Pharmaceutical Management Agency New Zealand 2003. *Annual Review* (www.pharmac.govt.nz).

Polis, B. 2001, *Only a Mother Could Love Him, ADD: Attention Deficit Disorder*, Seaview Press, Henley Beach.

Prosser, B. 2005, *Seeing Red: Critical narrative in ADHD research*, Post Pressed Publishers, Flaxton.

Prosser, B. and Reid, R. 1999, 'Psychostimulant Use for Children with ADHD in Australia', *Journal of Emotional and Behavioral Disorders*, vol.7, no. 2, pp.110–117.

Prosser, B., Reid, R., Shute, R. and Atkinson, I. 2002, 'Attention Deficit Hyperactivity Disorder: Special education policy and practice in Australia', *Australian Journal of Education*, vol.46, no. 1, pp.65–78.

Rappaport, J. and Buschbaum, M. 1980, 'Dextroamphetamine: its cognitive and behavioral effects in normal and hyperactive boys and normal men', *Archives of General Psychiatry*, vol.37, pp.933–943.

Reid, R., Maag, J.W. and Vasa, S. F. 1994, 'Attention Deficit Hyperactivity Disorder as a Disability Category: a critique', *Exceptional Children*, vol.60, no. 3, pp.198–214.

Reid, R. and Katsiyannis, A. 1995, 'Attention-Deficit/Hyperactivity Disorder and Section 504', *Remedial and Special Education*, vol.16, no. 1, pp.44–52.

Reid, R. 1996, 'Three Faces of Attention-Deficit Hyperactivity Disorder', *Journal of Child and Family Studies*, vol.5, no. 3, pp.249–265.

Reid, R., Reason, R., Maag, J., Prosser, B. and Xu, C. 1998, 'Attention Deficit Hyperactivity Disorder: a perspective on perspectives', *Educational and Child Psychology*, vol.15, no. 4, pp.56–67.

Reid, R., Hakendorf, P. and Prosser, B. 2002,'Use of Psychostimulant Medication for ADHD in South Australia', *Journal of the American Academy of Child and Adolescent Psychiatry,* vol.41, no. 8, pp.1-8.

Schachar, R. 1986,'Hyperkinetic Syndrome: historical development of the concept' in *The Overactive Child,* ed. E.Taylor, Blackwell, Oxford, pp. 19-40.

Shaywitz, S. and Shaywitz, B. 1988.'Attention Deficit Disorder: current perspectives' in J. Kavanagh and T.Truss Jnr. (eds.), *Learning Disabilities: proceedings of the national conference.* New Work Press, Parkton, pp. 69-523.

Slee, R. 1994,'Finding a Student Voice in School Reform: student disaffection, pathologies of disruption and educational control', *International Studies in the Sociology of Education,* vol.4, no. 2, pp.147-172.

Smelter, R., Rasch, B., Fleming, J., Nazos, P. and Baranowski, S. 1996.'Is Attention Deficit Disorder Becoming A Desired Diagnosis?, *Phi Delta Kappan,* vol. 77, no.16, pp.429-432.

Smyth, J., Hattam, R. and Lawson, M. (eds.) 1998, *Schooling for a Fair Go,* The Federation Press, Sydney.

Smyth, J. 2001, *Critical Politics of Teachers' Work,* Peter Lang, New York.

Stevens, G. 1981,'Bias in the attribution of hyperkinetic behavior as a function of ethnic identification and socioeconomic status', *Psychology in the Schools,* vol.18, no.1, pp.99-106.

Thomson, P. 2002, *Schooling the Rustbelt Kids: making the difference in changing times,* Allen & Unwin, Sydney.

Wakefield, J. 1992,'The Concept of Mental Disorder: on the boundary between biological facts and social values', *American Psychologist,* vol.47, no. 3, pp.373-388.

Wallis, C. 1994.'Life in Overdrive', *Time USA,* 18 July.

Vines, G. 1993. *Raging Hormones: Do They Rule Our Lives?* London, Virago.

World Health Organisation [WHO] 1993, *International Classification of Diseases (ICD-10),* World Health Organisation, Geneva.

Zametkin, A. 1989,'The neurobiology of attention-deficit hyperactivity disorder: a synopsis', *Psychiatric Annals,* vol.19, no. 11, pp.584-586.

Index